Edited by
CHRISTINE DEAN
HUGH FREEMAN

Community Mental Health Care

International Perspectives on Making it Happen

GASKELL &
The Centre for Mental Health Services Development

© The Royal College of Psychiatrists 1993

Published by Gaskell on behalf of the Centre for Mental Health Services Development.

Gaskell is an imprint of the Royal College of Psychiatrists, 17 Belgrave Square, London SW1

British Library Cataloguing-in-Publication Data
Community Mental Health Care:
International Perspectives on Making it
Happen
  I. Dean, Christine II. Freeman, Hugh
  362.2

  ISBN 0-902241-58-3

Distributed in North America
by American Psychiatric Press, Inc.
ISBN 0-880486-23-6

The publishers are not responsible for any error of omission or fact.

Printed in Great Britain by Redwood Books, Trowbridge, Wiltshire

Community Mental Health Care

International Perspectives on Making it Happen

Contents

Contributors

Piers Allott, Consultant, The Centre for Mental Health Services Development, King's College London, Campden Hill Road, Kensington, London W8 7AH

Paddy Cooney, Consultant, The Centre for Mental Health Services Development, King's College London, Campden Hill Road, Kensington, London W8 7AH

Tony Day, Consultant, The Centre for Mental Health Services Development, King's College London, Campden Hill Road, Kensington, London W8 7AH

Christine Dean, Consultant, The Centre for Mental Health Services Development, King's College London, Campden Hill Road, Kensington, London W8 7AH

Stephen Dorrell, MP, Financial Secretary to the Treasury, Treasury Chambers, Parliament Street, London SW1P 3AG

Ann Foster, Consultant, The Centre for Mental Health Services Development, King's College London, Campden Hill Road, Kensington, London W8 7AH

Hugh Freeman, Honorary Professor, University of Salford, and Honorary Consultant Psychiatrist, Salford Health Authority; 21 Montagu Square, London W14 IRE

Pat Holmes, Consultant, The Centre for Mental Health Services Development, King's College London, Campden Hill Road, Kensington, London W8 7AH

John Hoult, Consultant, The Centre for Mental Health Services Development, King's College London, Campden Hill Road, Kensington, London W8 7AH

David King, Leader of the Mental Health Task Force, Room 237, Department of Health, Richmond House, 79 Whitehall, London SW1A 2NS

Peter McGeorge, Consultant Psychiatrist, Mental Health Services, Design Implementation Review, 23 Essex Road, Mt Eden, Auckland, New Zealand

Roger C. S. Moss, Consultant, The Centre for Mental Health Services Development, King's College London, Campden Hill Road, Kensington, London W8 7AH

Mary O'Hagan, Consultant, The Centre for Mental Health Services Development, King's College London, Campden Hill Road, Kensington, London W8 7AH

Alberto Parrini, Psychiatrist, Mental Health Department, USL 9, Prato, Italy

Edward Peck, Consultant, The Centre for Mental Health Services Development, King's College London, Campden Hill Road, Kensington, London W8 7AH

Jan Pfeiffer, Psychiatric Centre Prague, Ústavní ulice, 181 03 Praha 6 – Bohnice, Czech Republic

Pino Pini, Psychiatrist, Mental Health Department, USL 9, Prato, Italy

Simonetta Gori Savellini, Professor of Psychology, Psychology Department, Florence University, Florence, Italy

Leonard I. Stein, Professor of Psychiatry, University of Wisconsin Medical School, Department of Psychiatry, B6\240 Clinical Science Centre, 600 Highland Avenue, Madison WI 53792, USA

Introduction: opportunities for change

DAVID KING

Where does change come from? In our society a number of factors produce change: new technology (e.g. the telephone and the aeroplane), competition in the high street, public demand for change, well informed articulate consumers, and more responsive providers. The latter two are the factors most likely to provide the incentive for change in our mental health services.

About 12 or 15 years ago, I thought that change could be achieved by replacing the Victorian hospitals which had induced dependency in their inhabitants and which had resulted in the removal of the mentally ill from society. However, I now consider that, although removing these hospitals is important, it is only one component in the move towards better services.

A factor which hinders change is that many of the professions are still training in the systems of the past, and not in the systems of the present. Each profession has its own professional territory and procedures, and this can make it difficult for them to collaborate and to work as a team. In addition to these divisions there is compartment-alisation of health care, social care, and housing. This can result in ridiculous situations, for instance professionals being unable to decide whether bathing someone is health care or social care. Some professionals do not like collaborating with users, carers, or the voluntary organisations in the delivery of services, and this hinders progress.

There are some optimistic signs – the Royal College of Psychiatrists is keen to find ways to improve the training of psychiatrists in a community mental health approach, and there are successful examples of teams that do work in an equal and responsible way, both among themselves, and in relation to their customers. Although improved training and team working would help in the improvement of service delivery, again it is only part of the solution.

The absence of management capability to effect change has been a problem in the past but now, with the advent of general management, this should not be the case. However, it is still regarded as a possible detriment to a manager's career to have worked in the mental health services, and this discourages many managers. Managing change is very complex and requires good managers; it is also a most exciting and rewarding area of work.

Although there does not seem to be the commitment to change which transformed the Victorian mental health services or which was responsible for the building programmes of the 1960s and 1970s, there does seem a commitment to change in some of the authorities working with the Centre for Mental Health Services Development (CMHSD), and this seems to be a time when things might happen. There are, in my view, sufficient resources to achieve it.

Service users are beginning to have an impact on the development of services. Most previous services recognised the importance of meeting the needs of individuals, but these were often words on pieces of paper. A crucial change is the beginning of recognition that service users are of equal status as professionals – this is something that never existed in the heyday of the large mental hospitals.

There is the growing understanding that professionals should be assessing and meeting the needs of people rather than selecting individuals for existing services. These needs are those which can be met by services: decent housing, treatment, meaningful activity, and so on. There is also a recognition that services need to be comprehensive and integrated, and be services which meet the whole range of people's needs, including social needs.

These changes are welcome and must result in better services for people with mental illness which should aim to develop the talents and abilities of users to the full; development and independence, information and education for people and their families and friends should be the aim of new services. Market research needs to take place into the needs of users of mental health services and how to meet them.

Operational research evaluating the services provided is also important. For instance, investigation of why the demand for acute beds goes up when the community teams are not on duty may result in practical solutions such as having the teams on duty for longer hours of the day. Research which investigates how the various elements of service work together for the benefit of users is currently absent.

In order to provide the right services for people, it is not enough to just close hospitals, to improve better inter-disciplinary working, or to just have committed, energetic, and effective management. We will only get it right if those components are concentrating on the needs of the individual user, finding the most cost effective ways of meeting them, and are involving consumers and their supporters in service design and testing their satisfaction with services.

The following chapters are by authors from different countries who have addressed these matters and have put together services that do aspire to consumer-orientated change and are integrated solutions. Contributions are from Dane County in the USA where a service has been up and working for 15 years for a community the size of a district, from New South Wales where the services for an entire population have been transformed in more recent times, from Prato in Italy where there is much community involvement, from Prague in the Czech Republic where the first courageous steps are being made, from Auckland, and from Birmingham in the UK. There are people who have achieved comprehensive services who have not reported their work. One of the valuable roles of the CMHSD could be to act as a focal point for people who have achieved change.

Although it is 20 years since the 1975 White Paper there has been little progress towards achieving that vision. I used to feel exasperated that change did not happen quicker but now I recognise it may take 20 more years to implement the 1975 White Paper. However, the drive and determination has to continue, otherwise people will do nothing for 17 years and try and do everything in the last three years. In order for the changes to be complete in 20 years the commitment has to start today.

1 The history of British community psychiatry

HUGH FREEMAN

It seems to be characteristic of some processes of social history that they follow not a linear, but rather a circular trajectory. Thus, the mentally ill in Britain came under the aegis of 'community care' in pre-modern times, as they still do today in most developing countries where public responsibility is limited to confining those cases who present a physical danger to others. The history of the parish church of Youlsgreave in Derbyshire, for instance, records a payment to the wardens for purchase of cord to bind a woman who was 'furiously mad', in the late 16th century. The Poor Law of 1601 clearly defined the responsibility of every parish to maintain those who were incapable of caring for themselves; this responsibility, though, was limited to people defined as 'settled' in the parish, and any who were not could be expelled from it. (The Community Care provisions of 1993 are perhaps uncomfortably close to this in some ways.) Before the mid-18th century, there was only one institution in England for the care of the insane, and none in the other countries of the British Isles. This was Bethlem (or Bedlam), which has been widely quoted as representing neglect, cruelty, and professional incompetence, although this reputation was not fully deserved (Allderidge, 1985).

The growth of humanitarianism during that century, particularly associated with non-conformist religious groups, led to the construction of a number of hospitals for the insane, either as independent institutions or associated with general hospitals. These were supported by subscriptions from the wealthier classes, but others were operated for profit, initiating the 'trade in lunacy' (Parry Jones, 1972). In many of them, care was little better than at Bethlem, and it was concern over this state of affairs which led the Quakers to establish the 'Retreat' at York, where the principle of Moral Treatment was first developed by William Tuke (Digby, 1985). This was to be an influential force in psychiatric care, not only in Britain but also particularly in

1

the USA. Although often suffering the wrath today of those who denounce the 'medical model', Tuke was in fact a tea merchant, but his ideas were fairly soon adopted by those doctors who were put in charge of the early asylums.

For complex reasons, the psychiatric annexes to voluntary general hospitals in England were all closed by the early 1800s (Mayou, 1989). As a result, any institutional care of the mentally ill was in specialised hospitals, set apart from the mainstream of medicine and nursing, for the next 150 years. The unfortunate state of 'lunatics' confined in poorhouses, prisons, private madhouses, or family homes – as well as those who were homeless or wandering – continued to be a humanitarian issue. An Act of 1808 gave permissive powers to the Justices of each county to build asylums, which would be paid for by local rates, but this development was slow. Since many of those admitted to the asylums were destitute, the responsibility for their costs came under the Poor Law, which was amended in 1834 to require relief to be provided only within institutions. For better or for worse, this largely ended a policy of 'community care' that had been operating for well over two centuries. It meant the construction of a huge national network of workhouses.

The ideology underlying this change continued to see Britain as an agrarian and mercantile society, although it had already become the world's first industrialised nation. As a result, the size of towns and cities exploded on a previously unknown scale, with mass migration into them both from the countryside and from Ireland. Their unregulated growth produced enormous public health problems, one of which was the accumulation of larger numbers of people disturbed by psychosis than had ever been known previously in any single community (Cooper & Sartorius, 1977). In 1845, the counties were required to provide asylums, and most of Britain's mental hospitals were constructed during the next 25 years, with a second wave in the 1880s.

However, the workhouses became filled with abandoned children, infirm elderly, and those disabled by physical or mental illness, and not with work-shy adults, as the 1834 Act had feared. The intention of the law was that all those identified as mentally ill should be transferred to asylums, but since care in the workhouses was cheaper, their transfers were often resisted by the Guardians who administered the Poor Law. However, neither this reluctance nor a high death rate – mainly from disease and neglect before admission – prevented the asylums from growing steadily in size. This was partly due to the increasing population, but more through the accumulation of incurable cases who could not be discharged to poor families, or to no family at all. The workhouses, overwhelmed with sick and disabled people, became obliged to build large 'infirmary' annexes, which were in fact embryonic general hospitals; this occurred particularly from the 1860s onwards. In 1890, the law regulating asylums and compulsory care was codified, in a 'triumph of legalism' (Jones, 1972); the rigid procedures and criteria this imposed meant that only people suffering from severe psychosis were likely to be admitted. The mental hospital system then largely remained unchanged for over 40 years, developing an institutional culture that was counter-therapeutic in many ways, partly through its close involvement with the Poor Law.

It is very significant in the development of British social policy that in 1875 the government began to pay a subsidy to poor law authorities of up to 25% of the cost of maintaining 'pauper lunatics' in asylums; this was the first direct involvement of the central government in responsibility for the financing of any social or welfare service. Historians with a Marxist orientation, such as Foucault (1963) and Scull (1977) have seen these developments in terms of 'social control' and the removal of unproductive members from the industrial proletariat. The perceived threat to public order posed by the mentally ill cannot be ignored, but humanitarian concern was at least as important; studies of the early asylum records (e.g. Walton, 1986) show that people were only admitted when those outside were unable to care for them any longer. Many of these cases also suffered from serious physical illness or neglect; often, they were in fact failures of 'community care'. The mental hospital system began on a wave of optimism and idealism, similar to that accompanying community care in our own times, but before long became overwhelmed by the tide of then untreatable disorder. As a result, the principles of Moral Treatment were mostly lost, but it would be wrong to accuse the system of 'failure' through applying the criteria of today (Berrios & Freeman, 1991).

World War I and its aftermath

One of the outstanding features of World War I was the large number of psychiatric casualties; the term 'shell shock' came to be used to describe most of these problems, after punitive methods had failed to control them and attempts to find organic lesions had proved fruitless (Merskey, 1991). Methods of combined physical and psychological rehabilitation were then developed, and a few psychiatrists who had become aware of Freudian theories were involved in these. This wartime experience had some subsequent effect, in that the management of neurosis was now seen as a legitimate part of psychiatry. A few out-patient clinics were opened, mainly in London, at which psychotherapy was available, and the Cassel Hospital provided the same for in-patients (Pines, 1991). In 1923, the Maudsley Hospital was opened by the London County Council as the first public psychiatric hospital operating outside the restrictions of the Lunacy Act. The Tavistock Clinic was also founded, as a centre for psychotherapeutic training and treatment. These developments were all localised and on a small scale, but they represented the beginnings of an approach to psychiatric disorder that was not centred on the mental hospitals.

These institutions, however, had returned to operating much as they did before 1914, and dissatisfaction with them led to the appointment of a Royal Commission, which reported its findings in 1926. Its views were progressive for the time, and it recommended that mental illness should be dealt with on modern public health lines. However, the legislation of 1930 was a compromise: voluntary admission to mental hospitals was made possible; offensive terms such as 'pauper lunatic' were abolished; and out-patient work by the medical staff of public mental hospitals was permitted. By 1936, 143 such clinics were operating, although little is known as to what actually went on in them; some had social workers attached (Freeman & Bennett, 1991). A number of mental hospitals also established admission units, where voluntary patients, in particular, would be segregated from the mass of chronic cases. These were some further modest steps towards caring for psychiatric disorder outside the now traditional closed institution.

Reform of the Poor Law in 1930 had brought the workhouse infirmaries under the control of local authorities, and more of these institutions then progressed towards becoming general hospitals in a modern sense. Many had 'observation wards' to which acutely ill psychotic patients were admitted under the Lunacy Act, and then transferred to mental hospitals, unless they recovered quickly. Some also had long-stay 'mental' wards, which contained a mixture of patients with dementia, chronic psychosis, mental retardation, and epilepsy.

World War II and its aftermath

With the approach of World War II and expectations of mass civilian casualties, a national survey of all hospital facilities in Britain revealed an alarming picture of incoordination, neglect, and generally inadequate provision. In response to this, the Emergency Medical Service rapidly established new hospital units, run by salaried specialists. The need to improve morale in the armed forces and among civilians, through hope of a better future, led to planning for a National

Health Service (NHS). However, this at first excluded mental hospitals on the grounds that the mental illness law would have to be reformed before they could be merged with others. In 1945, Aneurin Bevan decided that the only way out of the impasse into which negotiations had sunk was to nationalise all hospitals within a single administrative system (Webster, 1988). This would provide the secondary level of health care through specialists, while primary care remained the responsibility of general practitioners (GPs), and access to the specialists would normally be through them. Local authorities were to provide accommodation for infirm old people, mainly in the former workhouses, and staff to arrange compulsory admissions to mental hospitals – representing an embryonic social work service. However, since the NHS was only one of a number of measures (social security, public housing, child welfare, etc.) which constituted the Welfare State, it was no longer necessary for people to remain in mental hospitals (as they had often done up until then), mainly to receive free medical care, shelter, and maintenance. All these services were now available to them in the general community, and in the post-war period of full employment, all but the most seriously disabled could find work. Subsequent developments in community psychiatry are best understood in relation to this background.

By the late 1940s, the first effective physical treatments, principally electroconvulsive therapy (ECT), had come into general use in Britain. Their main effect in mental hospitals was to increase the rate of turnover, since severely depressed people no longer had to be cared for over months or even years, but admissions began to rise ever more rapidly, leading to serious overcrowding. Out-patient ECT was also an important development, in that it allowed some people with quite serious psychiatric disorders to be treated while continuing to live at home. A significant number of new doctors had entered into psychiatry since the war, and these tended to have a more active approach to the management of patients than had been usual among the previous mental hospital staff. At the same time, the evolution of therapeutic community concepts from the wartime work of Main & Maxwell Jones (1952) was one of a number of ideological changes which challenged the traditional habits and thinking of institutional psychiatry.

However, it was the discovery in the early 1950s of neuroleptics which provided an impetus for more fundamental changes. In 1955, the number of occupied psychiatric beds in England and Wales which, except for falls during the two World Wars, had been rising for over a century, showed a reduction for the first time – as it did in the USA, but not in other industrialised countries. This resulted from a combination of direct pharmacological effects, greater confidence among psychiatrists that people suffering from psychosis could be discharged earlier, and the new possibilities of treating patients with medication or ECT outside hospitals. By 1960, this fall in bed numbers had become so marked (Tooth & Brooke, 1961) that, two years later, a national Hospital Plan foresaw a rapid run-down of the mental hospitals and their replacement, although on a much reduced scale, by beds in district general hospitals (DGHs). By then, the introduction of antidepressants and tranquillisers had further increased the scope of drug treatment, both in general practice and in out-patient psychiatry, where the numbers seen grew rapidly.

Other developments that were to be important for community psychiatry occurred during the 1950s. Day hospitals began to be established, increasing the flexibility with which psychiatric treatment could be offered, and further reducing the use of hospital beds; (although in an opposite trend, the ageing of the population caused a greater demand for the in-patient care of dementia). The Mental Health Act of 1959 swept away a great deal of old restrictive legislation, allowing most psychiatric admissions to occur informally. The first hostels and therapeutic social clubs provided support particularly for discharged patients. In north-west England, some district psychiatric services developed from general hospital bases – former workhouse infirmaries – and ceased to use beds in the region's mental hospitals, thus providing a model for future changes (Freeman, 1960). Psychiatric nurses started to work with patients outside hospitals. By the end of the decade, locked doors were disappearing from psychiatric hospitals and wards, and traditional restrictive habits were being abandoned. The effect of all these changes, which probably occurred earlier in Britain than anywhere else, was to reduce greatly the rigid separation that had always existed between psychiatric in-patient care and the outside world. In spite of shortages of all resources (except mental hospital beds), there were widespread feelings of optimism about the way ahead. This began to be spoken of as 'community psychiatry', although the term did not represent any change in theoretical models. As with most developments in Britain, it consisted of a series of pragmatic responses to changes that mostly originated outside the mental health care system.

The 1960s and after

The 1960s was mainly a period of consolidating these same trends. Unlike the USA or the former West Germany, nearly all Britain's modest number of psychiatrists worked wholly or primarily within NHS hospitals, and because of the remarkable autonomy of the consultant's role, they could then pursue innovative schemes, provided these did not require spending much money. (This would hardly be possible in the 'reformed' NHS of today.) Since hardly any new hospitals were being constructed, the small amounts of capital available were used for alterations to the largely Victorian building stock. Local progress towards a more comprehensive service was achieved mainly by better integration between hospital-based psychiatry, local authority community services, and GPs (Freeman, 1963). Within the mental hospitals, rehabilitation and industrial therapy were developed, together with the beginnings of specialised services for the elderly, children and adolescents, forensic cases, and misusers of alcohol or drugs. All these in turn were to form their own links, as time went on, with community-based provision such as local authority facilities for old people or disturbed children. Home visits by all the professions became increasingly common, especially to evaluate patients before possible admission to hospital. There was growing emphasis on continuity of care for people from defined populations, whatever the nature or severity of their psychiatric disorder, thus avoiding wasteful bargaining between services or the passing of responsibility from one to another. Apart from an overall shortage of resources, the main problem, however, was the enormous variability of local authorities in their level of provision of community services; these were almost entirely local decisions, which central government – having refused to 'earmark' any grants for the purpose – could hardly influence. Also, by the end of the decade, the Western 'cultural revolution', beginning in Paris, saw the growth of antipsychiatry, which exposed some mental health services, particularly in large cities, to mainly political hostility.

Psychiatrists, even more than most other specialists in the NHS, began to see increasing numbers of patients first at home, on domiciliary visits. This arrangement had been designed for people who could not readily attend hospital out-patient clinics, and it was assumed that the GP would normally be present so that he/she could continue with treatment in the home. In practice, psychiatrists found that the initial evaluation of a case was often more effective in a patient's familiar surroundings, with relatives present, than in a hospital clinic. The attendance of GPs occurred to varying extents, but their place was taken increasingly by a social worker or psychiatric nurse. Medical visits to patients' homes later evolved in various ways – particularly in the work of crisis-intervention teams.

The 1960s were additionally marked by a strong divergence between the interpretation and implementation of community psychiatry in Britain and the USA respectively (Bennett & Freeman, 1991). The British version was one of developing services for defined communities, with emphasis on the needs of those most severely ill or disabled, and of integration of hospital with extramural care. The American policy, seen in the Kennedy legislation of 1963 and subsequent construction of comprehensive community mental health centres, focused on the goals of primary prevention and 'positive mental health', mainly through psychotherapeutic intervention in less severe conditions. In this latter case, the new form of care was not integrated with the work of state mental hospitals, where bed numbers were drastically reduced (Grob, 1991). The American approach is more accurately described as 'community mental health' than as 'community psychiatry'.

The 1970s and 1980s

The 1970s began in Britain with a rapid growth in public expenditure, although this was brought to a halt; first by the oil crisis of 1973, and then by financial restrictions in 1976. However, the building of new DGHs had at last gathered some momentum, and this resulted in a growing contribution to psychiatric in-patient care by general hospital units; in 1970, these had accounted for only 15.5% of admissions. In the first half of the decade, managerial reorganisation was seen as the key to efficiency in every major service: nursing, social work, local government, and the NHS all experienced this in turn, with very mixed results. In social work, a generic formula was imposed, virtually ending the special skills of psychiatric social workers; at the same time, all were made employees of the local authorities, with whom hospital psychiatric units now had to negotiate for a social work service. This 'integration' of the profession meant, in practice, the disintegration of mental health teams, where these had been established (Jones, 1979); the reorganisation had been carried out without any preliminary research or any serious inquiry as to whether they were likely to achieve the benefits claimed (Martin, 1984). Most psychiatrists came to believe that the consequences of this change were disastrous, and the overall quality of mental health care almost certainly suffered permanently as a result. The NHS reorganisation did not affect psychiatry more than other specialities, but the new managerial structure was seriously flawed and had to be changed again in 1982.

Although the officially approved direction of change for British mental health services had been clear since the late 1950s, there had so far been no comprehensive statement of national policy. After a preliminary publication in 1971, this eventually emerged as *Better Services for the Mentally Ill* (Department of Health & Social Security, 1975). Its declared aim was to establish a comprehensive service for each Health District (with an average 250 000 population in urban areas), based on a DGH psychiatric unit. The running down or closure of mental hospitals was not to be a primary objective, but only a consequence of better services being provided in this way, although the number of occupied psychiatric beds had in fact already fallen by 60 000. The NHS would continue to depend on local authority social services for such community-based facilities as sheltered accommodation and day centres. Target norms were laid down for each form of provision, including 0.5 hospital beds per 1000 population for general psychiatry, although it was clearly a long process to achieve this. Another significant development during the decade was the establishment of the Royal College of Psychiatrists in 1971, especially because of the highly organised national system of specialist training and examination which it instituted. The number of psychiatrists in post was already increasing rapidly, but it was now guaranteed that they would be of improving professional quality, which would in turn be reflected eventually in better national standards of mental health care.

Other professional cadres also grew significantly in number during this decade, including GPs, who continued to be responsible for managing the great bulk of less severe psychiatric morbidity. As psychiatry was starting to assume an important place in the undergraduate medical curriculum, it could be expected that younger GPs at least would be better equipped to undertake this function.

Finally, the 1970s saw the emergence of community psychiatric nursing as a speciality with its own training; it grew rapidly, partly because of the general disappearance of psychiatric social workers. The first 'out-patient' nurses had been appointed in 1954 at Warlingham Park Hospital, Croydon. Their duties included visiting out-patients who had failed to attend or who needed to be seen between attendances, supporting in-patients who had been discharged, helping to find jobs or accommodation for them, and being available to give advice at out-patient clinics or therapeutic social clubs. One of the reasons for this development was a severe national shortage of mental health social workers. Subsequently, as the in-patient sector began to shrink, psychiatric nurses began to be appointed to work entirely outside hospitals, although from a variety of bases and with differing sources of referral. These numbers began to grow in the 1970s, and then even more sharply in the 1980s; although largely unplanned, this increase outstripped the growth of all other groups of mental health personnel. Community psychiatric nurses (CPNs) came to fall into one of two main groups: those working within a psychiatric multidisciplinary team (which could be based in a psychiatric hospital, a general hospital psychiatric unit, or a mental health centre), and those working in a primary health care setting. The second of these arrangements was encouraged by the fact that many psychiatrists also began to spend part of their time in general practice facilities, but this had the effect of breaking up the mental health team. Views varied greatly about the optimal way for community nursing to be organised, and this was associated with increasing ambiguity about how the responsibility for patients should be shared and about the respective accountability of CPNs to doctors or to their own professional managers (Rawlinson & Brown, 1991).

The first phase of growth of community psychiatric nursing was associated with the trend to extramural management of schizophrenia, which itself was encouraged by the extensive use of depot neuroleptics (Freeman, 1981). CPNs came to take on an essential role in ensuring that those schizophrenic patients who could not be relied upon to attend a hospital clinic regularly would in fact continue to receive regular injections; this could be in their own homes, at health centres, at day centres, in hostels, in group homes, etc. The growth of the service was also associated with the development of post-qualification training courses for psychiatric nurses.

After a few years, specialised CPNs came into being, working exclusively with one type of patient: psychogeriatric, mentally handicapped, forensic, those requiring behavioural therapy, etc. Specialisation greatly improved the quality of care that could be offered to each group, but at the same time increased costs in a way which became alarming when real resources for the mental health services were scarcely growing overall. As a national service, community psychiatric nursing by trained staff seems to be unique to Britain, but provision is still at a varying level in different parts of the country – although less so than that of social workers.

Depression is the most common psychiatric disorder, both in the community and in the GP's surgery, although anxiety-related symptoms often predominate in new episodes of illness. In Britain, most depressed people are seen by their GP during the illness, although their complaints are often somatic and the psychiatric disorder may not be diagnosed; family doctors still vary widely in their ability to detect these conditions (Tantam & Goldberg, 1991). The most common method of management in primary care is by psychotropic medication, particularly antidepressants; until the mid-1980s, benzodiazepines were widely prescribed for anxiety, but their use is now restricted to short-term treatment. Psychological treatments such as counselling and cognitive therapy have become more prominent in recent years, but are largely dependent on the availability of suitably trained staff. Although GPs are well placed to provide a continuous service to people in the community with chronic disorders, particularly schizophrenia, this has not happened effectively on any large scale; this responsibility has nearly always remained directly with the specialist psychiatric services. In spite of the development of alternative service models such as crisis intervention, most initial contacts for psychiatric care are still with the GP, who refers directly to a psychiatrist when necessary. Apart from the presenting severity of the patient's condition, the most common criterion for referral is probably failure of response to the initial treatment. In the early years of the NHS, most GPs were either in single-handed practice or small partnerships, usually working in their own homes or converted accommodation (such as old shops); the trend since then has been towards larger groups and practice in purpose-built health centres. There has also been a considerable growth in the activities of other health professions within primary care; these include several (CPNs, counsellors, clinical psychologists, social workers) who are wholly or partly concerned with the care of psychiatric patients.

For Britain, the 1980s may be said to have begun in 1979, with the return of a new 'conviction' Government and dissolution of the 'liberal consensus' which had influenced social policy since World War II. Although the framework of mental health objectives remained outwardly unchanged, major differences of emphasis soon emerged. There was certainly a policy dilemma, in that over 70% of mental health expenditure – which in turn was some 20% of NHS expenditure (Office of Health Economics, 1989) – was taken up by hospital costs. While this limited the growth of community-based services, mental hospitals were supposedly not to be closed until a better service was available to replace them. In fact, a notable acceleration in the process of hospital run-down and closure could soon be observed, and this often aroused alarm, both among mental health professionals and among the relatives of patients with more severe disorders, particularly schizophrenia. It was not so much the resettlement of long-stay hospital residents which caused this concern (although these arrangements were not always what might have been expected from government statements), but rather the inadequacy of resources to care for patients already living in the general community who had long-term disabilities or recurrent episodes of decompensation. At the same time, structural unemployment was rising to levels not known since the 1930s, so that the chance of paid work for anyone with a psychiatric handicap virtually disappeared.

As a proportion of Gross Domestic Product, UK health expenditure remained the lowest among advanced industrial countries during the decade, while NHS funding persistently failed to increase in line with the true rate of inflation. Circumstances, therefore, were not propitious for a major reorientation of mental health services – as was required by the rapid shrinking of mental hospital resources – and these financial problems were compounded by disagreement over objectives.

Whereas psychiatrists saw 'community psychiatry' as the provision of high-quality professional care on a local basis, with the least possible disruption to patient's normal lives, some other professionals, users' representatives, and local politicians – in a re-run of 1960s' anti-psychiatry – sought either to deny the existence of psychiatric illness altogether, or the need for anyone to be in hospital on that account.

The decade (if one may expand it at the other end to 1991) was one in which administrative changes, policy statements, and proposals for reorganisation (some implemented and some not) came thick and fast. The Mental Health Act 1983 was to some extent a 'lawyers revenge' for that of 1959; it had no relevance to the overwhelming majority of people with psychiatric disorders (Jones, 1988). A report by the independent Audit Commission (1986) was strongly critical of the state of 'community care', as the House of Commons Social Services Committee (1985) had been. They had recommended that no psychiatric patient should leave hospital without a comprehensive care plan that had been agreed between the various services involved. The Griffiths Report (Griffiths, 1988) advised that local authorities should have the responsibility for all 'community care', but was unclear about the distinction between care and 'treatment', the latter remaining the province of the NHS. The NHS & Community Care Act 1990 implemented some of the Griffiths proposals, but others were postponed until 1993 because of their implications for local authority budgets. As from 1991, individual care plans became mandatory for patients discharged from hospital, and a Mental Illness Specific Grant was the first direct subvention from the government to local authorities which could be used only for community mental health services, although the case for it had been strongly argued 30 years earlier (Titmuss, 1961). Also in 1991, the most fundamental reorganisation of the NHS since its inception in 1948 seemed to make financial considerations paramount, while the separation of many hospitals or other services into independent trusts posed a threat to the planning and integrative efforts that had patiently been pursued over many years. Both these trends seem likely to have unfavourable implications for the development of community-based psychiatry.

The 1980s also saw a rapid increase in the number of mental health centres operating in Britain; while there was much diversity between these (and some were not very different from DGH units, except for the absence of beds), indications emerged that many were following American trends of the 1970s (Good Practices in Mental Health, 1991). They were tending to concentrate on patients with less severe neurotic personality or situational problems, at the expense of those with serious, long-term disorders. CPNs were also affected by the same tendency (Wooff *et al*, 1988) – an ironic development, since this service had partly come into being because of the general abandonment of these clients by social workers after the Seebohm reorganisation.

The 'key worker' and 'case worker' concepts were also introduced, with both roles being taken at times by the same individual, but an unresolved issue was how to reconcile the needs identified by such a person with the constraints of limited (and sometimes shrinking) resources. Similarly, the 'multi-disciplinary team' has often been seen as fundamental to community-based work, but without clarifying the way in which the special skills, status, and legal responsibilities of the consultant psychiatrist fit into that framework. Crisis intervention by such teams has been advocated as a more effective alternative to conventional methods of providing psychiatric services; it might be particularly suitable for areas with high rates of psychiatric morbidity (Dean & Gadd, 1989).

Unresolved issues

Freeman & Bennett (1991) described the British view of community psychiatry as an "eclectic, non-ideological, and largely atheoretical discipline ... open to and capable of absorbing ideas or data from any school, provided that these are found pragmatically to be capable of reducing disease, distress, or disability". While this national understanding of the term owes more to the biological than to any other model, "it is equally open to psychodynamic concepts or to such sociological ones as social support and social networks".

In this development, since the end of World War II, such pragmatic questions as how the needs of the relatively small number of people who have severe psychiatric disabilities can be managed have tended to be converted by some into an ideological issue – all care within a hospital by professional staff being labelled as 'oppressive'. From a different point of view, the need to protect the community from the few mentally disordered individuals who show disruptive or dangerous behaviour is often denied by those responsible for planning or managing services, mainly because the facilities required to deal with those cases are expensive, particularly in staff time. British community psychiatry has shown that it can replace many, but perhaps not all, of the functions of the traditional mental hospital, which was often the place of last resort for individuals with multiple and undifferentiated problems.

Grob (1991) pointed out that, in the USA, a reform movement which began with concern about the condition of people with long-term disorders in mental hospitals ended by setting up a completely new care system, which in fact offered nothing to that group; with the run-down of state hospitals, they were left worse off than ever. In Britain, the possibility remains that the same process could occur, although a well evaluated solution for those who need constant nursing care is the hospital-hostel. The first unit of this kind was established in a large old house, adjacent to the Maudsley Hospital in south London. An uncontrolled study (Wykes & Wing, 1982) showed that patients attained a better social adjustment there, compared with those of similar clinical status who had remained in hospital wards, while the cost was somewhat lower. In south Manchester, there has been detailed evaluation of a similar unit, in an old house quite separate from the hospital campus. There, two groups of patients were matched for chronicity, clinical features, and problem behaviour; they had been ill for an average of 12 years, had prominent florid symptoms, and needed 24-hour nursing care. After two years, those in the hospital-hostel had fewer defect symptoms, had acquired more skills, and had spent their time more usefully; they much preferred life in this setting to being in hospital. Nursing costs were higher in the hostel unit, but its 'hotel-type' maintenance costs were much lower (Hyde *et al*, 1987). It would seem feasible to establish several such units for any population, forming a network around a hospital base, each caring for a different kind of patient needing long-term care. So far, however, no such arrangement exists, in Britain or elsewhere.

Although a unit of this kind can operate well in ordinary domestic accommodation, it needs permanent staffing at the level of an acute hospital ward; managers whose 'performance' is measured by a balance-sheet tend to be unable to unwilling to accept this. At a more modest level, larger numbers of those chronically disabled by psychiatric disorder need long-term 'asylum' – shelter, protection from exploit-ation, and whatever degree of rehabilitation is possible. The care of this group requires a coordinated policy between the NHS, social services, and voluntary organisations, but little attention has been given to the problem, and virtually no controlled comparison has been made of possible facilities that might replace the mental hospital for this purpose (Wing, 1990).

A final problem that has emerged in recent years is how to accommodate the views of users of community psychiatric services. The British tradition in these matters has been a paternalistic one, starting with the aristocratic patrons of charitable hospitals, and followed by the work of such public health pioneers as Snow, Simon, and Chadwick. The service developments after World War II followed a similar direction, in which psychiatrists and medical civil servants played the leading roles. With the growth of consumerism and of more egalitarian trends in British society, however, it was to be expected that professional views of this kind would be less prevailing. Britain has had a long tradition of voluntary effort in the mental health field, beginning with the establishment in 1863 of the Mental After-Care Association, which has continued to provide a number of residential homes for discharged patients in the Greater London area, with a limited period of stay. In 1948, it was the only one of the existing voluntary organisations which did not amalgamate to form the National Association for Mental Health (NAMH). Essentially an alliance of professionals and interested volunteers at the national level, NAMH lobbied for better services, offered pilot training services (e.g. for social workers and residential care staff), published information on both facilities and general issues, and provided advice to members of the public. At a local level, relatives of the mentally ill were more active, and the emphasis was mainly on providing care facilities, such as day centres and hostels. In 1972, the organisation changed its name to MIND and took on a much more 'radical' philosophy, resulting in the eventual departure of most of the mental health professionals from its councils.

Partly as a consequence of this change (in which hostility to psychiatric hospitals became increasingly strident), but also through a feeling that the problems caused by schizophrenia were not adequately recognised, a new organisation was set up by relatives of people suffering from that disorder. The National Schizophrenia Fellowship (NSF) has provided both a means of mutual support for these families and a strong voice against the premature running down of hospital facilities, while the community-based service that is supposed to replace them still remains incomplete. Two organisations – the Mental Health Foundation, and Schizophrenia: A National Emergency (SANE) – have been primarily concerned with obtaining funding for psychiatric research, although SANE now offers a telephone advice service.

A Department of Health discussion paper (1990), on planning district mental health services, urged health authorities to obtain views from the main users of services, particularly as to which activities they regarded were key indicators of good performance. It is far from clear, however, how this can be done in a genuinely representative way. Community-based mental health services, including the contribution of primary care, may have contacts with over 20% of the population, and among these millions of people, there are likely to be diverse views.

References

ALLDERIDGE, P. (1985) Bedlam: fact or fantasy? In *The Anatomy of Madness, Vol II* (eds W. F. Bynum, R. Porter & M. Shepherd), pp. 17 – 33. London: Tavistock.

AUDIT COMMISSION (1986) *Making a Reality of Community Care.* London: HMSO.

BENNETT, D.A. & FREEMAN, H.L. (1991) (eds) *Community Psychiatry: The Principles.* London: Churchill Livingstone.

BERRIOS, G. E. & FREEMAN, H. L. (1991) (eds) *150 Years of British Psychiatry.* London: Gaskell.

COOPER, J. E. & SARTORIUS, N. (1977) Cultural and temporary variations in schizophrenia: a speculation of the importance of industrialisation. *British Journal of Psychiatry*, **130**, 50 – 57.

DEAN, C. & GADD, E. (1989) An inner city Rome treatment service. *Psychiatric Bulletin*, **13**, 667 – 669.

DEPARTMENT OF HEALTH & SOCIAL SECURITY (1975) *Better Services for the Mentally Ill* (command 623). London: HMSO.

DEPARTMENT OF HEALTH (1990) *Planning District Mental Health Services.* London: HMSO.

DIGBY, A. (1985) *Madness, Morality & Medicine: a History of the York Retreat.* Cambridge: Cambridge University Press.

FOUCAULT, M. (1963) *Madness & Civilization.* New York: Vintage Books.

FREEMAN, H. L. (1960) Oldham & District Psychiatric Service. *Lancet*, *i*, 218 – 221.

—— (1963) Community mental health services: some general and practical considerations. *Comprehensive Psychiatry*, **4**, 417 – 425.

—— (1981) Long-term treatment of schizophrenics. *Comprehensive Psychiatry*, **22**, 94 – 102.

—— & BENNETT, D. H. (1991) *Community Psychiatry.* London: Churchill Livingstone.

GOOD PRACTICES IN MENTAL HEALTH (1991) *Community Mental Health Teams.* London: GPMH.

GRIFFITHS, R. (1988) *Community Care: Agenda for Action.* London: HMSO.

GROB, G. N. (1991) *From Asylum to Community.* Princeton: Princeton University Press.

HOUSE OF COMMONS SOCIAL SERVICES COMMITTEE (1985) *Community Care with Special Reference to the Adult Mentally Ill and Mentally Handicapped.* London: HMSO.

HYDE, C., BRIDGES, K., GOLDBERG, D.P., *et al* (1987) The evolution of a hostel ward: a controlled study using modified cost benefit analysis. *British Journal of Psychiatry*, **151**, 805 – 812.

JONES, K. (1972) *History of Mental Health Services.* London: Routledge & Kegan Paul.

—— (1979) Integration or disintegration of the mental health service. In *New Methods of Mental Health Care* (ed. M. Meacher). Oxford: Pergamon.

—— (1988) *Experience in Mental Health: Community Care and Social Policy.* London: Sage.

JONES, M. & JONES, M. (1952) *Social Psychiatry.* London: Tavistock.

MARTIN, F.M. (1984) *Between the Acts.* London: Nuffield Provincial Hospitals Trust.

MAYOU, R. (1989) The history of general hospital psychiatry. *British Journal of Psychiatry*, **155**, 764 – 776.

MERSKEY, H. (1991) Shell-shock. In *150 Years of British Psychiatry* (eds G.E. Berrios & H. L. Freeman), pp. 245 – 267. London: Gaskell.

OFFICE OF HEALTH ECONOMICS (1989) *Mental Health in the 1990s.* London: OHE.

PARRY JONES, W. (1972) *The Trade in Lunacy.* London: Routledge & Kegan Paul.

PINES, M. (1991) The development of the psychodynamic movement. In *150 Years of British Psychiatry* (eds G. E. Berrios & H. L. Freeman), pp. 206 – 231. London: Gaskell.

RAWLINSON, J. W. & BROWN, A. C. (1991) Community psychiatric nursing in Britain. In *Community Psychiatry* (eds D. H. Bennett & H. L. Freeman). London: Churchill Livingstone.

SCULL, A. T. (1977) *Declaration: Community Treatment and the Deviant – A Radical View.* Englewood Cliffs, N.J.: Prentice-Hall.

TANTAM, D. & GOLDBERG, D. P. (1991) Primary health care. In *Community Psychiatry* (eds D. H. Bennett & H. L. Freeman). London: Churchill Livingstone.

TITMUSS, R. (1961) Community care: fact or fiction. In *Proceedings of the Annual Conference of the National Association for Mental Health.* London: NAMH.

TOOTH, G. C. & BROOKE, E. M. (1961) Trends in the mental hospital population and their effect on future planning. *Lancet, i,* 710 – 713.

WALTON J. K. (1986) Casting out and bringing back in Victorian England: pauper lunatics. In *The Anatomy of Madness, Vol II.* (eds W. F. Bynum, R. Porter & M. Shepherd). London: Tavistock.

WEBSTER, C. (1988) *The Health Services Since the War, Vol I. Problems of Health Care. The National Health Service Before 1957.* London: HMSO.

WING, J. K. (1990) The functions of asylum. *British Journal of Psychiatry,* **157,** 822 – 827.

WOOFF, K., GOLDBERG, D. P. & FRYERS, T. (1988) The practice of community psychiatric nursing and mental health social work in Salford: some implications for community care. *British Journal of Psychiatry,* **152,** 783 – 792.

WYKES, T. & WING, J. K. (1982) A ward in a house: accommodation for 'new' long-stay patients. *Acta Psychiatrica Scandinavica,* **63,** 315 – 330.

2 Creating change: a case study

LEONARD I. STEIN

Bringing about change starts with an idea, but what happens to the idea once it is exposed to public scrutiny is greatly influenced by the environment surrounding it. If the idea is congruent with the traditions, ideology, and practice of the environment in which it is spawned, it will be protected and encouraged to grow and bear fruit. If, on the other hand, the idea is contrary to or inconsistent with these traditions, its life is much more hazardous, its rate of growth slower, and its chances of growing strong enough to bear fruit much less.

This chapter presents such an idea for change. It is based on the philosophy that community services for mental health that are supported by public funds should have, as their highest priority, a service for the most severely mentally ill patients. Strange as it may seem, this was contrary to the practice of most community mental health centres operating in the USA from their inception in the mid-1960s, until the 1980s. These centres, mainly developed to treat people with severe mental illness, were actually staffed by professionals trained to do dynamically orientated psychotherapy, appropriate for a much healthier population. These centres operated as large out-patient psychotherapy clinics, so that to change them to focus on severely ill patients would have required modifications – including the type of treatment, working hours, and hierarchical relationships between staff members that were inconsistent with their mode of current practice. Furthermore, treating people with chronic mental illness in the community would demand greater tolerance on the part of the community for those people, and would even necessitate a change in how the patients themselves coped with stress. Thus, it is not surprising that this effort to bring about change ran into formidable obstacles.

The case study in this paper describes change in the mental health system in Dane County, Wisconsin, USA.

Dane County, Wisconsin, USA

Dane County has a population of 340 000 people: approximately 200 000 live in Madison, and the rest in small towns and on farms. Approximately 1500 people suffering from chronic mental illness who receive care from the publicly funded system have been identified. The county has used its normal funding mechanisms creatively in order to develop a broad-based, multi-agency system of care for this chronic mentally ill population. It is important to note that the system is not especially well funded to run an optimal programme, spending less than the national average per capita. The services could be more fully developed if more funds were available, but the programme is succesful because the money is spent extremely efficiently. (Specific funding strategies will be described in a later section of this chapter.)

The services as they existed in 1974

In 1974, the major provider for mental health services to the severely mentally ill of Dane County was one of Wisconsin's two State mental hospitals which was geographically located in the area. This 650-bed hospital had a number of long-stay residents from the county, but most of its activity was with the population of revolving-door patients; there was little in the way of services for them, once they were discharged from the hospital. The Community Mental Health Center, being primarily an out-patient psychotherapy clinic, offered them little. It did provide, however, medication-evaluation and prescription services for those patients who came to the clinic to receive them, as well as a socialisation group one evening a week, once again for those willing to come for that session. There were a few other services, for example recreational, vocational, and social work, for patients motivated enough to find them and meet the requirements for entrance. This mix of hospital and community services operated in an uncoordinated, non-collaborative fashion. Together, they comprised a non-system of mental health care, where a few patients got more than they needed, many got less than they needed, and some got nothing at all. Patients became lost in this non-system, and no-one felt obligated to look for them; a major problem with it was that it was episode-orientated rather than being designed to provide continuous care. This non-system not only failed the patient, but also undermined the potential effectiveness of the professionals working in it.

Events that influenced change

There were several events that made change possible, ranging from new legislation which changed the State Mental Health Act, to a change in leadership at the Community Mental Health Center.

In 1971, the State of Wisconsin enacted a new Mental Health Law with the intent of changing the non-system into a coordinated system of care. An amendment to this legislation in 1973 required every county to plan for and provide (or purchase) services for the mentally ill; importantly, this mandate also included paying for in-patient services. Before this legislation, the State paid for in-patient services only in the State hospitals. Subsequently, funding for both hospital and community services would be provided by the State to each county on a formula basis, with the expectation that the county would contribute a minimum of 9% in matching funds. In essence, the legislation decentralised control of mental health services from the State level to local control at the county level. Previously, there were separate funding streams from the State for hospital and community services respectively: these separate streams were quite inflexible, and it was almost impossible to shift money from one to the other. In 1974, approximately 70% of the public mental health funds were being used to support institutional care, while 30% was supporting care in the community. However, as a consequence of the legislation, the county now had all the funds, and could allocate them in any way it saw fit. This allowed for great flexibility and for a reallocation of money from hospital to community care.

The other event which facilitated change in Dane County was the change in leadership of the Community Mental Health Center: in 1974, both its Executive Director and Medical Director left. The new Executive Director, a young social worker, Robert Mohelnitzky, and the new Medical Director, myself, had a different vision about how mental health centres should operate. We thought that their priorities were unconscionable ones – that most of their resources were being directed towards people with relatively minor illnesses, while those with serious illness were largely neglected. While nearly every other area of medicine operates on the basis that people who are most in need of care should get it first (the leftover resources being used for people with lesser problems), it was our perception that mental health services in the USA practised this concept in reverse. Further, both of us believed that the severely mentally ill were, first and foremost, citizens of our community who happened to have a psychiatric disability. They had a right to live in the community, in a stable fashion, and to receive their services in the community. We felt that we should not have to beg the community to let these citizens live there: it was the community's responsibility to allow its citizens to live wherever they could. We believed that the goals of the Mental Health Center were, firstly to help persons with severe mental illness live stable, meaningful lives of decent quality, and secondly to provide the support and education to the community which would allow that to happen.

To have the Center reach this goal would necessitate major changes in its activities. It would have to change from being an out-patient psychotherapy clinic to a multiprogramme one that made serving the needs of the seriously mentally ill its highest priority. We were determined to bring this change about.

Services as they exist today

Before considering the barriers to change that confronted us, it might be helpful to describe what the product of that change looks like today.

Crisis Resolution Services

The Mental Health Center of Dane County provides a 24-hours-a-day, seven-days-a-week Crisis Resolution Service that has a mobile capacity to go to the client if the client is unable to go to the Center. The Center also staffs a 24-hour telephone service which works closely with the mobile crisis team. Together, the mobile crisis team and the crisis telephone unit form an integrated Crisis Resolution Service (Cesnik & Stevenson, 1979). The telephone service receives calls from all parts of the community, including people in need, families, police, and other mental health providers, as well as the emergency rooms of the general hospitals. It provides direct help and consultation, often acts as an information bank for other mental health professionals, and refers calls which require immediate face-to-face attention to the mobile crisis team.

By definition, crisis teams operate in the midst of crises: the person in crisis, his/her family, and the community are often all emotionally upset. Therefore, the crisis staff have to be prepared to deal with resistance and conflict. A shopkeeper might demand that we get someone off the street in front of his shop when the patient has a legal right to be there. A patient or family member may come in demanding admission to hospital when this is not clinically indicated. At times, admission is indicated and used, but more often, careful assessment together with the development of a definite treatment plan, permits successful out-patient resolution of the crisis, with minimal risk. An important part of this process is the availability of staff 24 hours a day, to reassess the crisis plan continually, as required.

From its inception, the crisis team was developed with a strong out-patient orientation. Its job is to work with both the patient and the community to stabilise the immediate crisis, and then to continue providing whatever service is necessary, until either the crisis is resolved or a transfer to ongoing treatment can be arranged. As such, the crisis team in Dane County is different from many emergency services which act only to assess the need for immediate admission, but are not designed to assume any responsibility for true crisis resolution. The crisis team is at the centre of the Dane County mental health system, and considerable effort has gone into making sure that it is effective.

The team consists of five full-time equivalent (FTE) telephone workers, eight FTE crisis workers, a secretary, 20 hours per week of staff psychiatrists' time, and 30 hours per week of psychiatric residents' time. The experience of the crisis team over the last 17 years of its operation has reinforced its conviction that most people who come into a crisis service or into an emergency room do not need admission. What they do need is a careful assessment, the development of a clear treatment plan, and monitoring to make sure that this plan is put into practice. With such monitoring, the team can assess whether their ongoing plan is effective, and modify it as needed.

Often, the person in crisis is someone who is already in the system, receiving treatment for a psychiatric illness. In such cases, the crisis team has immediate access to the person's clinical records and treatment plan. The availability of good clinical records is critical to an accurate assessment of the risks, as well as to the development of effective treatment options. Records include a history of past suicidal or assaultive behaviour, some information about the person's support system, a description of what has helped in the past, the medication history, and often a specific plan to deal with any crisis that might arise. If such information is not available, the person's case manager is contacted for further information and for joint treatment planning with the crisis team.

Mobile Community Treatment programme

The Mobile Community Treatment (MCT) programme was designed specifically to serve the most difficult-to-treat patients in the system (Stein & Diamond, 1985). This programme is a direct replication of the Training in Community Living (TCL) programme (Stein & Test, 1980; Weisbrod *et al*, 1980; Test & Stein, 1980). The patients targeted for this programme suffer either from schizophrenia or from other mental illnesses, and have a history of repeated admissions. Since these patients often resist coming in regularly to receive services, they need assertive outreach. They often are not compliant with medication, so that this also requires a specialised approach. Many need to have some structure of daily activities provided, and most are poor at monitoring themselves, so that they require regular monitoring. They tend to have frequent crises. Since their social network is absent, overwhelmed, or tenuous, they need professional psychological support. Finally, they have significant deficits in coping skills and are not able to negotiate the system; thus, they require a great deal of case management services.

The MCT programme was developed to help severely ill people with schizophrenia to live in the community, to decrease their need for psychiatric hospital care, and to enhance their quality of life. Much of it is orientated towards providing help with the normal tasks of daily living, teaching coping skills so that, over time, patients can accomplish things on their own, and providing a support system for those who have little in the way of social support or human contact. Much of the treatment involves practical activities such as helping a patient maintain his/her apartment, going shopping with him/her for groceries, or teaching the patient how to use a washing-machine at a local laundrette. Verbal interaction between staff and patients is important, but it is easier for many of these patients to form relationships when staff spend time helping them meet their concrete needs, than it is when contact is restricted to talk in a therapist's office. Two key parts of the programme are assertive outreach and a strong case management system; this latter part assures that patients' needs are being met, that problems are recognised early in their development, and that patients do not drop out of treatment.

The MCT programme operates two shifts a day, from 8.00 a.m. until 10.30 p.m., seven days a week; night-time emergency back-up is provided by the Mental Health Center's Crisis Resolution Service. The MCT programme currently has nine full-time personnel, plus a programme manager, a programme secretary, and approximately 30 hours of psychiatrists' time a week, to treat 150 patients. Experience has convinced the staff that its patient:staff ratio is too high: these patients need intensive services if they are to survive in the community. To work effectively with the difficult-to-treat patient, a patient:staff ratio of 10:1 would be optimal. The MCT staff can dispense medication seven days a week, hand out spending money on a daily basis, arrange for food vouchers at restaurants, go grocery shopping, or accompany the patient to a new voluntary job. Over time, some patients become relatively stable and need less intensive services; they may come in once a week to make contact with staff, or every two weeks for a depot antipsychotic injection. Even these relatively stable patients, however, need close monitoring in order to prevent decompensation and readmission.

One important priority of the MCT programme is to work closely with other parts of the patient's support system. For example, many patients also have a welfare worker concerned with them, or receive visits from the Visiting Nurse Service. Sometimes, the waitress in a restaurant where the patient eats every day is in a better position to help monitor and detect early signs of crisis than are the MCT staff members, who see the patient less often. Employers and landlords are much more willing to be helpful when they receive support and assistance from the MCT staff. Finally, families – even those which have been considered resistant to family therapy – often play an important and positive part in the patient's treatment, when a psycho-educational approach is being used. Confidentiality and autonomy have to be respected when working with these extended support systems, but helping the patient to coordinate the other people and services in his/her life is a critical factor in maintaining stability.

The patients followed by the MCT programme are frequently in and out of crisis, often have extraordinary needs, and require staff who are more available than any doctor could be. Therefore, a case management system based on a team rather than on an individual is used to provide continuity of care and to protect individual members of staff from the burden of sole responsibility. It is important for the entire staff to know all the patients, to be kept up to date on their current status and treatment plans, and to share responsibility.

Both formal and informal mechanisms have been developed to ensure that communication and coordination within the team function smoothly and that patients are not lost through the cracks in the system. Every staff/patient contact, from a patient's brief daily visit for medication to contact in an emergency room following a suicide attempt, is described in a daily logbook, so that staff members starting their shift can scan all the events of the last several days. During the daily afternoon shift-change meeting, every patient in the programme is reviewed at least briefly, with both day and evening staff present. Every patient has a treatment plan: some involve daily staff contact, while others require much less. As a result, patients who have missed appointments, or who need a special service or some kind of follow-up can all be identified, and specific staff assignments made for them. Once a week, a longer staff meeting allows time for treatment planning on new or problematic patients. While only those staff working on a given day are present during daily shift changes, the schedule allows most staff to attend the weekly meeting, to ensure that everyone is kept aware of any problems and is actively involved in the treatment-planning process. All staff, from the secretary to the psychiatrist, actively share information, so that the entire team functions as a coordinated unit. While coordination of the team takes time to implement, it is critical if the programme is to be effective.

Yahara House

The Yahara House programme is Dane County's psychosocial rehabilitation unit for chronically mentally ill adults. As with other clubhouse-type programmes, this one has adopted many of the principles developed at Fountain House, New York City, USA (Beard *et al*, 1982). It has a strong vocational emphasis and provides basic skill training, social support, and a way of structuring time. People who attend its activities are considered members, and the programme is arranged such that it cannot function without the real services that the members provide. Telephones are answered, meals are cooked, minor maintenance of the building is undertaken, and even some of the outreach to members who have not been attending is done by other members. Professional staff are responsible for providing structure and supervision but, once the culture is established, even much of this falls on the members themselves to maintain. Thus, professional staff become free to spend much of their time providing either case management or outreach services, both of which are essential to minimise drop-out from the programme and to maintain members' stability in the community.

The programme operates seven days and four evenings a week, and for holidays such as Thanksgiving and Christmas as a replacement for the extended families and support system that many of the members lack. It is dedicated to providing people who have severe and persistent mental illness with effective and comprehensive services which can assist them to lead more independent, healthy, and fulfilling lives in the community. The programme works with those patients who are relatively stable, have at least some motivation, and are able to tolerate group activities. It is organised into units, each with an area of responsibility: all the units are connected with a range of vocational opportunities, including transitional employment positions (TEPs) in the community. The basement unit is responsible for meals – arranging menus, buying food, cooking and serving it, and cleaning up after the lunches and dinner that are served to approximately 70 members a day. The first-floor unit runs the telephone and reception area, keeps track of the attendance of members, and does much of the paperwork required to operate the Yahara House programme. The second-floor unit puts out both the daily and weekly newsletters, makes posters, undertakes publicity for special events, and puts out special educational booklets such as one on the value of work. The second-floor unit also produces a weekly video programme which is broadcast on the city public-access cable television channel.

An additional part of the programme is the medical unit. Historically, there has been some tension between those clubhouse programmes which operate on the basis of a rehabilitation model, and those using a medical model. In most programmes, treatment services such as monitoring and prescribing psychotropic medication are disconnected from the clubhouse, and are provided by a separate staff at a separate site. Yahara House has worked instead to integrate medical services within the rehabilitation framework. Information about medication is shared between medical staff and members: the emphasis of the medical unit, as in the other units of the programme, is for members to gain a sense of expertise and competence. Members not only learn about their medication and their illness, but are also encouraged to acknowledge and share their own expertise about different medication, side-effects, how this affects them, and what techniques they have learned to deal with symptoms of the illness.

Adult Clinical Services and Meds-Plus

The Adult Clinical Services programme is an out-patient clinic which provides services to many different kinds of patients. Approximately 40% have chronic schizophrenia: many of these do well without elaborate services – they neither want nor need more than brief contact, support, and monitoring. Patients come in every two to four weeks to see the Meds-Plus nurse for medication monitoring, under the supervision of a psychiatrist. They are seen initially for an evaluation by a psychiatrist, and at one- to three-monthly intervals thereafter, depending on need. For some of these patients, more intensive involvement might become too intrusive and might disrupt a rigid but precarious stability. Other patients come in once every two to four weeks for supportive counselling, medication monitoring, and prescription renewal. Some group activities, some case management services, and some crisis intervention services are available from the patient's regular therapist, but if a patient temporarily requires more intensive services, the Crisis Resolution Services assist.

It is important to reassess the needs of these patients on a regular basis. A patient who has been stable with minimal support might need more intensive help if his/her parents become unavailable or if his/her support system changes in some other way. Other patients who were not interested in vocational rehabilitation might become much more open to this kind of help as they grow older. Other programme units and other kinds of assistance need to be available for the patients who require more than this minimal level of service. At the same time, in a system with scarce resources, we cannot afford to take up a slot in a more expensive programme if minimal support is all that is needed or wanted.

The three services described above are among many others available in Dane County today. However, it is clear that their mode of operation and staff relationships are different from those that operate in a traditional out-patient psychotherapy clinic.

Barriers to change

To get from an out-patient psychotherapy clinic to what has been described above required overcoming barriers which may be unique to this particular case study. Nevertheless, when one attempts to bring about change in an environment that is resisting it, there is little doubt that barriers will be erected, and for change to succeed, specific strategies must be developed.

Resistance by the professional staff

Virtually the entire professional staff of the Mental Health Center of Dane County previously were mental health professionals trained to do psychotherapy; they liked doing it and were largely uninterested in changing. The first thing the Executive Director and I decided to do was to expand our crisis service so that it could be more effective, and get it involved in stabilising crises, rather than just making an evaluation and disposing of people in crisis. The latter often led to hospital admission, whereas the former would work towards helping people remain stable in the community. Fortunately, our budget that year allowed for the employment of some new staff members, but according to personnel policy, we first made those positions available to the existing staff. That none volunteered was no surprise to us, and thus we hired people who wanted to do that kind of work.

The first major problem with the staff arose when we decided to develop a continuing care team, to target a group of patients frequently in hospital care who were living unstable, chaotic lives and revolving in and out of the hospital at a rapid rate. To respond to the needs of that group of patients, we decided to develop the MCT programme described above. The work of this progrmme was very different from sitting behind a desk, having clients come into the office for psychotherapy. Since staffing this unit necessitated using current staff, we had to reduce the size of our out-patient psychotherapy service. We asked the current staff for volunteers.

The first response of the staff was to send a delegation to caution us that the community would not tolerate reducing the out-patient psychotherapy services. They warned us that such an action would bring the community's ire down on our heads, and suggested that we were asking for big political trouble. We considered what they said, but we also took into consideration the Center's reputation at that time. The families of people with serious mental illness thought we were less than useless. The police, who picked people up who were acting bizarrely in the streets and who came to us for help, were continually frustrated by not receiving what they wanted. In the past, when the administrators of the Center went to the County for annual budget meetings, they were continually harassed by the County Board to justify their budget. The Board was not convinced that the Center was particularly useful. So its reputation was a poor one to begin with, and there did not seem to be much to lose by moving in this new direction. We advised the staff that we were willing to take the gamble.

We again asked for volunteers for this new mobile outreach team that was to be developed, but it was no surprise that there were none. Following accepted personnel policy, the most recently hired staff were then chosen to be reassigned to this programme: they were faced with the decision of either accepting this or leaving the Center. In fact, all the reassigned staff entered the programme, but immediately began looking for other jobs. A few found that they really enjoyed what they were doing, but most found other jobs and left. This provided vacancies for people to be hired who would be interested in doing this kind of work. Within a relatively short time, the programme was enormously successful, and stabilised a large group of people who had been living unstable and chaotic lives and who were high users of hospital beds. The hospital money saved through this reduction of hospital use was used to develop another programme to stabilise another group of patients to save more money to continue the process. Thus, over 15 years, the clinic has changed from an out-patient psychotherapy clinic to a multiprogramme clinic.

Another example of a barrier encountered with the professional staff follows. One Sunday at 3.00 a.m., the police brought a patient into the crisis resolution unit. The unit staff, on getting his name, checked the records and found that he was indeed a clinic patient. They attempted to telephone the psychotherapist responsible for his care to get some information about the patient. However, this number was an unlisted one, so the psychotherapist was unreachable. The next morning there was a memo on my desk from the manager of the crisis resolution unit, advising me that it would be very helpful if his unit could have the telephone numbers of the Center's staff. Their intention was not to ask the staff to come in, but to just be able to telephone them to get information about their clients if a crisis arose. As Medical Director, I sent out a memo describing the situation, and asking for telephone numbers. I made it clear that we had no intention of asking anyone to come into the Center out of hours, nor to require them to not go on leave or to stay home at all times. Numbers were received from staff working in the newly developed units; but there was also a memo, signed by all the psychotherapists who still remained, saying that they worked from 9.00 a.m. to 5.00 p.m., Monday to Friday, and that they felt the rest of the time was their own, so that no telephone numbers were given.

Was it that these people were uncaring? I knew many of them *were* caring people. However, these remaining psychotherapists were all social workers or psychologists who, in their training, had been socialised differently from doctors and nurses, who are accustomed to accept responsibility for their patients' care 24 hours a day, and also expect that they might be called at night. The Executive Director and I explained the situation to the Board of Directors and asked them if they would be willing to make it a contingency of employment that telephone numbers of all staff members were made available. They agreed, and another memo was sent out, asking for either a number or a letter of resignation. We received telephone numbers.

At the present time, however, professionals are employed who enjoy their work, are committed to working with seriously ill patients, and find that they get a great deal of satisfaction from doing so in the kinds of programmes that have been developed.

Barriers from community members

In the USA, when members of the public are asked whether they believe that psychiatric patients should live in the community like the rest of us, there is generally an affirmative response. However, when there is an attempt to develop a group home, the neighbourhood generally organises to resist such a development. This is usually referred to as the NIMBY (Not In My Back Yard) syndrome. Thus, we had to work hard to get community acceptance in neighbourhoods where we were developing group homes or other types of special living arrangements.

In one case, we were going to build a small apartment unit on an empty site. This was quite an unsightly place, and we thought the neighbourhood would accept the idea of replacing it with a well kept and attractive small apartment unit. The community, however, continued to be resistant, because of their fear of psychiatric patients. We met them many times, until one night was the turning point. One of the them stood up and said, "I have been living in this neighbourhood for ten years, and none of you have known that I have a serious mental illness". That was a courageous thing for this woman to do, and it did much to sway the community in our direction.

One other thing happened that night which I think pushed the neighbours over the edge to acceptance. I told them that if we built that unit we would carefully choose the people living in it, and we would be available to them 24 hours a day, seven days a week, in case of any problems. I further told them that if we did not build the apartment unit, it was certain that someone else would, and in all likelihood it would be rented to university students. When they heard this, they all voted to give permission to build.

We now have two apartment buildings and several group homes. We have had virtually no difficulty with neighbours, and we have made an effort to be good neighbours ourselves. It is ensured that the buildings are well maintained and that the grounds are kept neat. We in fact try to do more than what is ordinarily expected so that any prejudices which might still exist can be overcome. In the neighbourhoods that have had these facilities for some time, we have successfully overcome these prejudices. When the community get to know the mentally ill patients as people, it becomes clear that the differences between them are generally small.

Problems with agencies

In our community there are many agencies funded with public monies that are there to serve the citizens of the community. Since we view the clients we work with as, first and foremost, citizens of the community, it was natural for us to go to these agencies and ask for their help. An example is the Visiting Nurse Service, which sends nurses to people's homes to help with their health care. We explained to them that our clients could benefit from this care. Their response was the same as we got from virtually every agency we went to: "We have no experience with psychiatric patients, and we are concerned that we may say the wrong thing, and something dreadful might happen – really, you would be better off without us".

We told them we understood how they felt and that we would have one of our nurses accompany their nurses until they felt comfortable going by themselves. In addition, we would remain available at any time to help with any problems that arose. They agreed to try it. Now, there are quite a number of psychiatric patients being served by the Visiting Nurse Service. They go to patients' homes, give depot injections, provide support, and give information to us. One visit to a mentally ill person's home is often more useful in determining functioning than many visits to a clinic.

However, not all agency contacts worked out so well. We approached another agency we thought could be helpful to our patients, and told them that we had some citizens who happened to have a psychiatric disability, and who could use their help. They told us they had no experience with psychiatric patients and "would probably do more harm than good". We told them we understood, and offered them the same support we offered the Visiting Nurse Service. They still refused. We informed them that as a United Way agency, they were prohibited from discriminating against anyone, including those with a psychiatric disability. They informed us that only 15% of their budget came from the United Way, and thus in essence were telling us that they would rather give up 15% of their budget than have to work with our patients. We then told them that the City of Madison has an ordinance which does not permit discrimination, and that we would take them to court. As with every agency to whom we threatened a court action, this agency then agreed to work with our patients.

Some of the agencies, however, remained so passive – aggressive in serving our clients that we dropped them; it was easier for us to do the work ourselves. However, many of them who got to know the patients as persons noted that they were indeed contributing something valuable, and these have become an important part of the service system. If we had not felt so strongly about our patients' citizens' rights, we would not have pushed as hard as we did, including the threat of court action. Had we not pushed hard, these agencies that are now part of the system would still be shunning psychiatric patients. It is important to note, however, that gaining and keeping agency cooperation requires more than a threat. There must be a willingness to provide education, support, and constant availability to them.

Patients' resistance to change

Our new programme targeted patients who were frequent users of hospital care, revolving in and out at a rapid rate. Many of them had, in fact, learned a maladaptive coping strategy – when they became anxious, they would do something to get back into hospital because in the past that was all that was available to them. Some would scratch or even lacerate their wrists and go to the emergency room of the general hospital, saying they felt very suicidal. Some would commit minor crimes, such as breaking a window or ordering food at a restaurant and then walking away and not paying for it. They would subsequently tell the police that they were mental patients, and the police would take them to hospital rather than to jail. They learned that these kinds of behaviour would get them back into the safety of an institution.

We had to help them learn more adaptive ways of coping with problems, and had to show that community services and supports could be more helpful to them than the hospital had been. Simply telling them this was not enough; they had to learn it by experience. This meant that when our service was called to an emergency room for somebody who had cut their wrists, we would go there and see if he/she was really suicidal or was hurting psychologically and desperately looking for help. If it was the latter, as it was in most cases, we would spend a lot of time with the person, helping to work through the current problems. After this patient was taken out of the emergency room, we would continue to work with him/her.

The doctors at the hospital were at first amazed at what we were doing, saying, "You are taking a suicidal patient out of the hospital". We told them that the person really did not want to die and was not suicidal, but needed help working through problems that were making him/her anxious. Furthermore, these problems could be best handled by working directly with the patient in the community. We further pointed out that wrist cutting was this patient's way of asking for help, and that we were going to try to give that help in a different way – one that we thought would be much better than the old way of simply admitting the patient. If the latter was done, then housing would often be lost or, if he/she had a job, that might be lost as well, and tenuous relationships with people would be disrupted; thus, taking the person back into the community would be a much more helpful way of handling the problem.

Some patients learned to give up their old maladaptive coping strategies quickly, while others did not change their strategy for quite some time. We learned that a consistent approach was important, and that if we admitted patients inappropriately, we would just be reinforcing maladaptive coping strategies.

Barriers to dissemination

Early in the process, when our work began to gain some recognition, it was not unusual for people to tell us that our work was interesting, but not adaptable to their own situation. They stated that we could do it here in Madison, Wisconsin, USA, but that where they lived, the situation was different, and it could not be done there. For years, we heard that Madison was a special place, with special people, an inference that somehow our psychotic patients were less psychotic and less problematic than other psychotic patients, plus many other reasons why we could do it and they could not. However, now that this model is being practised in many parts of the world as well as in many parts of the USA, including difficult, inner-city areas, little is heard of that view. What finally happened was that a growing number of places implemented the programme, and the number was sufficient to form a critical mass. When that critical mass was reached, it was as if a switch was turned on, and the view began to be expressed that if this model was not being followed, then a first-class service was not being implemented.

Another possible barrier was pseudo-implementation – places that continued to do what they had always done, but simply changed the name of the service. For example, the name of the out-patient psychotherapy clinic might be changed to an assertive community treatment team, while the staff still sat in their offices with appointment books, waiting for clients to come and see them.

Current problems

We still have a long way to go, and what is particularly frustrating at the present time is that with so much more to be accomplished, our funding is shrinking, and it is difficult to maintain the service. This may be a result of 12 years of a federal administration that has had a conservative funding policy towards disenfranchised people. Another reason, which may be very important to keep in mind as a caution for those systems moving in the same direction, is that when a system gets away from bricks and mortar, it becomes more difficult to justify its need for money to politicians. It is easy to point to a building that is beginning to fall apart and convince them that money is needed to take care of the problem. It is much more difficult to find something palpable in a community-based system that will capture their attention. Thus, it is important to establish a strong advocacy group of citizens to keep pressure on politicians, so that funding levels will be maintained.

Conclusions

Let me summarise what sustained us through this change process and which continues to sustain us now. First and foremost, we had an ideology that the clients we were working with are citizens of the community, and that they had a right to be in the community and to receive services there. Secondly, we felt it was important to translate that ideology into a goal for the severely mentally ill person: this is to help the person live a stable life of decent quality in an environment which affords that opportunity. Thirdly, we had a strategy for accomplishing the goal: this was that the community must be the primary locus of care, and that a broad approach to care must be used. The approach must include everything that is necessary to help achieve the goal, with attention paid to physical health, social support, social services, housing, finance, and so on. Lastly, we knew that in all our actions, we had to keep our eye on the defined goal noted, and that every decision we made had to be on the basis of whether it would help us advance towards that goal. Whenever times were difficult, we reminded ourselves of a saying: "Never doubt that a small group of dedicated individuals can change the world; indeed, that's all that ever has".

References

BEARD, J.H., PROPST, R.N. & MALAMUD, T.J. (1982) The Fountain House model of psychiatric rehabilitation. *Psychosocial Rehabilitation Journal,* **5**, 47 – 59.

CESNIK, B. & STEVENSON, K. (1979) Operating emergency services. In *New Directions for Mental Health Services, No. 2* (ed L.I. Stein), pp. 37 – 43. San Francisco: Jossey-Bass.

STEIN, L.I. & TEST, M.A. (1980) Alternative to mental hospital treatment, I. Conceptual model, treatment program, and clinical evaluation. *Archives of General Psychiatry,* **37**, 392 – 397.

——— & DIAMOND, R. (1985) A program for difficult-to-treat patients. In *New Directions for Mental Health Services, No. 26* (eds L.I. Stein & M.A. Test). San Francisco: Jossey-Bass.

TEST, M.A. & STEIN, L.I. (1980) Alternative to mental hospital treatment, III. Social cost. *Archives of General Psychiatry,* **37**, 409 – 412.

WEISBROD, B.A., TEST, M.A. & STEIN, L.I (1980) Alternative to mental hospital treatment, II. Economic benefit-cost analysis. *Archives of General Psychiatry,* **37**, 400 – 405.

3   The Sydney experience

JOHN HOULT

This chapter describes some research which was done in Sydney 12 years ago, how this research was then taken up into a State-wide system of care, and finally, the system of care which we want to achieve and the principles needed to make it effective.

For most of the 200 years since the British settled in Australia, the pattern of mental health services followed that of Britain. After an early phase of moral treatment in the mid-1850s, large mental hospitals similar to Britain's had been built by the late 19th century. In Sydney, this remained the major resource – in fact, almost the only one – for the care and treatment of the mentally ill until 1960. In that year, allegations of cruelty and neglect in one of these mental hospitals provoked a Royal Commission, which found them to be correct. The State Government subsequently spent large sums of money to upgrade the mental hospitals, and (following the British lead) to commence building psychiatric units in general hospitals. At the same time, psychiatrists began the process of deinstitutionalising patients from the long-stay wards, and of not allowing acute patients in the admission wards to become institutionalised.

Table 3.1 shows what happened subsequently. Since 1962 (the peak year for the number of people resident in mental hospitals) the State population has increased by almost 50%, the number of people resident in hospitals (both mental hospitals and general hospital psychiatric units) has fallen from 9000 to 2274, while admissions – which increased from 13 826 to a peak of 27 339 in 1980 – reduced to 21 689 in 1990. However, although the patients are no longer in the mental hospitals, the staff still are; the number of staff increased from 5000 to 7000 during the decade 1965–75, and were still at that level a decade later.

By the mid-1970s, a fragmentation of services had also developed. The mental hospitals, the general hospital psychiatric units, and the

TABLE 3.1
New South Wales: mental health statistics

	1965	1975	1990
New South Wales population	4.17m	4.88m	5.83m
Residents (mental hospitals and general hospital units)	12 421[1]	7426[1]	2285
Residents per 1000 population	2.98	1.52	0.39
Admissions (mental hospitals and general hospital units)	15 689	23 628	21 689
Admissions per 1000 population	3.76	4.84	3.72

1. Includes approximately 3000 intellectually handicapped people.

community mental health centres (which had been established a few years before) were all under separate administrative authorities and there was little or no linkage between the three. Furthermore, the general hospital units and community mental health services discovered a new clientele who had not sought service previously. People with neuroses, personality disorders, marital and family problems, and problems of living now came to seek help; gestalt therapy and transactional analysis swept into vogue. It was much more rewarding dealing with articulate people with relationship problems than with chronically mentally ill patients who had no conversational skills. The mentally ill were offered depot injection clinics, half a day each week in a group with an occupational therapist, or some attention from the most junior nurse on the team.

By the late 1970s, new problems were emerging. Many mentally ill were in cheap, unregulated, private boarding houses, and episodes of exploitation in these were being publicised. Many more were at home with relatives – mainly parents – receiving inadequate support, and these people were beginning to unite and become vocal in their protests.

In the Community Mental Health Centre in which I was working in northern Sydney, we were also becoming aware that all was not well, and that something needed to be done about it. I visited England and the USA, looking for good ideas. The most relevant ones seemed to me to be Dr R. D. Scott's Barnet Service in North London (in particular, his approach to separating the symptoms of mental illness from the behavioural disturbances associated with family reactions), and Dr Paul Polak's Service in south-west Denver, where acutely mentally ill patients were cared for and treated singly in the houses of private citizens, who were paid for providing a bed for this purpose.

I returned to Sydney determined to try to implement some of these ideas. By chance, there was an enquiry into mental health services soon after my return: one of the members of the enquiry team told me that money was available from the Commonwealth Government to research such projects. Although I had not done research previously, I was willing to do it in order to get money to start a project, so I decided to apply for a grant.

On reading the scientific literature in order to make sure I was getting the methodology right, I came across the early reports of the work by Stein *et al* (1975). The type of service they had provided seemed likely to work for us in Sydney. Their methodology was also good, and so I decided to replicate their study.

Our research project began in 1979 in northern Sydney; a more detailed report of it has been published elsewhere (Hoult, 1986). In brief, 120 consecutive people who presented or were presented to their local admission unit (Macquarie Hospital, a state mental hospital) were randomly allocated to two groups. The only exclusions were those aged below 16 years, or over 65 years, or with a primary diagnosis of drug or alcohol dependence, organic brain disorder, or mental retardation; however, people who were suicidal, dangerous, or violent *were* included in the project.

Those allocated to the control group received standard hospital care and follow-up, that is they were seen by the hospital duty doctor, almost all were admitted, and after an average of three weeks' stay, they were referred to one of the six community mental health services in the area for follow-up.

People allocated to the experimental group received a different treatment strategy. They were seen at the hospital by a member of a special community treatment team and its psychiatrist. After assessment, either the patient was admitted under the psychiatrist's care, or, more likely, was taken home or to some other community setting by the team member, and treatment of the illness was commenced there. The supervision was intensive at first: patients would be seen sometimes three or four times a day, and visits to them could last several hours. Much time was spent in planning treatment with the patient and with relatives or other members of the patient's social network. The community treatment team was available to patients and relatives 24 hours a day, and they were encouraged to contact it whenever necessary. If the patient could not stay at his/her home, the team assisted in finding alternative accommodation, such as a boarding house, and supported the patient there. As quickly as possible, the patient was expected and encouraged to become responsible and to resume normal duties. As patients became less psychotic, the team supervision and help lessened, but for those with a chronic, severe illness, the team remained involved on a regular, sometimes even daily, basis.

TABLE 3.2
Number of admissions to psychiatric hospitals or clinics during the 12-month study

	Experimental (*n* = 53)	Control (*n* = 47)
None	32 (60%)	2 (4%)
1	17 (32%)	21 (45%)
2	2 (4%)	17 (36%)
3	1 (2%)	5 (11%)
4 +	1 (2%)	2 (4%)

Since the project lasted for 12 months, the community treatment team and its psychiatrist were responsible for the care of the experimental group patients throughout that time. The team consisted of seven staff – three nurses, two social workers, a psychologist, and an occupational therapist – who were rostered on two shifts per day, seven days a week. Three staff worked from 8 a.m. to 4 p.m., two from 3 p.m. to 11 p.m., and one of the latter remained on-call at home throughout the night. Additional rates were paid for overtime and call-back work.

All patients in the study were evaluated by an independent team, which was responsible to a research psychologist. Initially, most of the patients were suffering from a functional psychosis. The results of the assessment after 12 months showed that most experimental group patients were not admitted, whereas almost all of the control group patients were (Table 3.2). Half the control group were readmitted to hospital in the study period, which is similar to other published studies, whereas only 8% of the experimental group were readmitted. Those experimental group patients who were admitted to hospital mostly stayed less than a week, whereas the control group had much longer stays (Table 3.3). In fact, over the 12-month study, the control group patients spent an average of 53.5 days in psychiatric hospitals or clinics, while the experimental group patients spent an average of

TABLE 3.3
Length of stay in psychiatric hospitals or clinics during the 12-month study

	Experimental (*n* = 53)	Control (*n* = 47)
Not admitted	32 (60%)	2 (4%)
Less than 1 week	14 (26%)	11 (23%)
1–2 weeks	0 (0%)	6 (13%)
3–4 weeks	3 (6%)	5 (11%)
5–6 weeks	3 (6%)	8 (17%)
7–10 weeks	0 (0%)	4 (9%)
11–15 weeks	0 (0%)	6 (13%)
16 weeks or more	1 (2%)	5 (10%)

8.4 days. The experimental group also had fewer symptoms at follow-up. Both patients and relatives preferred community treatment, and those who had experienced it were more positive about it than the control group were about standard hospital care and follow-up.

A cost-effectiveness study of the project was completed by health economists (Cass & Lapsley, 1983). This showed that over the 12-month study, the average treatment cost (public and private, direct and indirect) for each patient in the experimental group was A\$ 4489, and for each patient in the control group was A\$ 5669, that is standard hospital care and aftercare cost 26% more. The cost of treatment in the mental hospital alone for the control group was approximately equal to the cost of the total treatment of the experimental group.

In summary, our study showed that our model of community care resulted in fewer admissions and fewer bed-days, produced a better clinical outcome, was preferred by patients and relatives, and was considerably cheaper.

Our research results were in line with other controlled studies which have been completed elsewhere in the world (Braun *et al*, 1981; Keisler, 1982). Consistently, the results of these studies show that community-orientated care gives outcome results equal to or better than hospital-orientated care. When the community-orientated care is poorly resourced, the results show no significant difference, but when it is adequately resourced, the results favour community care. It is significant that there is no instance in all the published studies where hospital-orientated care comes out better.

So often, research in this field leads nowhere, but a number of mental health staff in Sydney, including Dr Alan Rosen, were determined not to be content with just one small area of the city operating this way. The opportunity came when there was yet another enquiry into mental health services; the previous one had not resulted in any appreciable action, but now homelessness was becoming apparent among the mentally ill.

In Britain, I have heard many people talk about homelessness of the mentally ill being a consequence of deinstitutionalisation, but research in both New York (Miller, 1985) and Sydney (Teesson & Buhrich, 1990) has shown that this is not the case. Patients deinstitutionalised from long-stay wards into community residences do not become homeless; rather, it is the non-institutionalised patients who become homeless. In a recent study of the largest shelter for homeless men in Sydney, a random sample showed that 26% of the men suffered from schizophrenia. Of the 22 men in the sample with this diagnosis, only three had had any appreciable continuous length of stay in hospital; most had had multiple short admissions, while some had not even been admitted at all (see Fig. 3.1). Furthermore, even though many of them had been going in and out of hospital for many years, it was not until 1981 – 82, when a housing shortage occurred in Sydney, that they became homeless. Thus, it is not the patients from the back wards who become homeless; rather, it is those from the admission wards, who are discharged after a short hospital stay because they are much improved.

In 1983, a number of clinicians proposed to this latest enquiry that the organisation and the principles of care used in our research project should be extended across the State. The enquiry accepted this proposal, and reported that services in New South Wales should be set up accordingly, with the target group being the seriously mentally ill. The enquiry's report acknowledged that there would not be unlimited money for implementing its recommendations: it advised that 'seeding' money should be given to set up good community services in one area; these should then reduce the use made of the mental hospital, freeing resources which could be transferred to another area, where the same process would in turn have an impact on the hospital, freeing further resources, and so on. Although extra money was needed for seeding funds, the process should be self-funding after that, and should be affordable.

The report led to uproar. The health unions claimed there would be massive dumping of patients in the streets and that the whole business was just a cost-cutting exercise. In spite of this, the Government

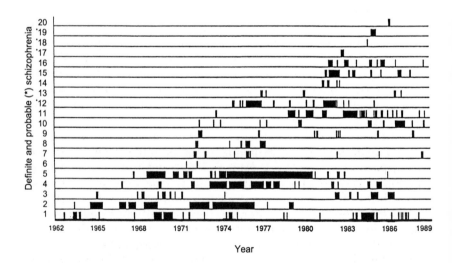

Fig. 3.1. Psychiatric hospital admissions for the 22 men diagnosed by the psychiatrist as having definite or probable schizophrenia (two subjects were never admitted)

did go ahead, and improved community services did eventuate. Many factors were important in this. Some examples will illustrate the fact that clinicians can influence the outcome of process of change. Early on, a group of clinicians met and decided that they should try to influence the decision-makers in the Health Department unit which would be implementing the report. This group met regularly, and because it knew what it wanted and kept lobbying for this, it was able to have considerable influence on the way services were set up. Equally as important, the service in northern Sydney which led the way has remained true to its goal, and is still a model for other services to emulate. It often happens that an innovative service collapses after a few years, as its original staff move on; this has not happened in northern Sydney because Dr Rosen and others have remained in the area and improved the service. Those who did leave northern Sydney did so to start up the new way of working in other areas and, in spite of sustained opposition, they have persevered and enabled the model and its principles to take root.

By 1988, all of northern Sydney, some parts of southern and western Sydney, and a few rural areas had changed over to this new way of organising and running their services. However, a State Government election was due and, during the campaign, the health unions switched their allegiance from the governing Labor Party (their natural allies) to the opposition Liberal Party, because the latter had promised to stop implementing the report. When the Liberals won the election, they stopped the programme and held yet another enquiry into mental health services. However, this enquiry's report, while recommending that a building programme be undertaken in our mental hospitals, also recommended that the improvement of community mental health services should be continued. What in effect happened was that the Labor Government programme continued under another guise. Although some new wards have been built, the overall operating costs in the mental hospitals have continued to be squeezed; the money saved has been 'ring-fenced' and used to set up new community services such as crisis teams and day centres.

These ideas are now becoming the accepted way of working in many parts of Australia. The Royal Australian & New Zealand College of Psychiatrists, which a few years ago was critical of the new initiatives, now deems it important for trainee psychiatrists to work in such services. Through persistence, we have been able to change the focus from a hospital- to a community-orientated service.

Research has been important in making the change: the results of the original study gave confidence that this approach was the most effective one. However, the criticism was made that this study had been undertaken in a relatively affluent part of Sydney by a specifically

TABLE 3.4
*Public Admissions from area to admission ward
(Ryde/Hunters Hill Crisis Team)*

Year	Admissions
1983	201
1984	217
1985	210
1986[1]	133
1987	109
1988	101
1989	90

1. Crisis team commenced June 1986.

chosen project team, and that the result would probably not generalise to less affluent areas and routine services. Consequently, in 1987, research was carried out into a routine crisis service in a middle-class area of Sydney: the Ryde/Hunters Hill Crisis Team (Reynolds *et al*, 1990). The results (Tables 3.4 and 3.5) show that this team was in fact also able to reduce the number of admissions and bed days of patients from its area. Furthermore, these results have been maintained; this area of 104 000 people continues to have about 100 admissions per year to public psychiatric beds, and on average uses only about five such beds for its adult population. This study also asked 55 patients and relatives their opinions about the service; the responses were similar to those of the original research. Eighty-eight per cent of patients were pleased they were not admitted, 80% were satisfied with treatment from the crisis team, and 85% thought the care and treatment from the crisis team was better than previous treatment. Eighty per cent of relatives thought the patient was helped by the

TABLE 3.5
*Bed days used by patients from area in admission ward
(Ryde/Hunters Hill Crisis Team)*

Period	Bed days
July–December 1984	1570
January–June 1985	2036
July–December 1985[1]	915
January–July 1986[2]	1806
July–December 1986	662
January–June 1986	690
July 1987–December 1988	2113

1. Nurses strike in this period.
2. Crisis team commenced in 1986.

crisis team, 84% were satisfied with the treatment from the crisis team, and 86% thought that the care and treatment the patient received from the crisis team was better than previous treatment. It seems that routine services can carry out this type of service and get results similar to the original project team, and that this will not increase the burden on families.

What lessons have been learnt from this experience that have wider application?

Have clear goals

Lack of clarity among staff as to who are their target groups and what are the tasks to be done for them can be a considerable problem. People with psychiatric problems can be divided into three groups (Fig. 3.2).

Firstly, there are those with 'serious mental illness'(SMI): people with psychoses make up perhaps three-quarters of this group, while the remainder have mixed diagnoses but a disabled lifestyle, similar to that of individuals with psychoses. This group is relatively small, but its members have a high level of need.

Secondly, there are people with other diagnosable psychiatric disorders, the largest group of whom suffer from depressive and anxiety neuroses. These people undoubtedly suffer from their symptoms, but as a group, they are more likely to be functioning better than the first one, and are more likely to know how to seek help.

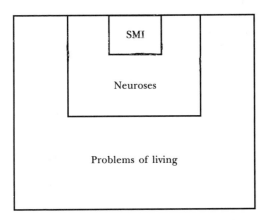

Fig.3.2. The patient population

The third group is a large one – 'the worried well'. These are people without a diagnosable illness, but who have relationship problems, family problems, or lack of self-fulfilment. They are often highly motivated to be helped and can often improve considerably with such help.

Since there are not enough resources to treat everyone, who should be targeted? Most services resolve this problem by taking whoever comes through the door, but this means that the most vocal, motivated, and cooperative patients will be treated, while the unmotivated and uncooperative – including most of those with serious illness – miss out. Whichever way the choice is made, someone will have to lose out. Unless a service targets a particular group, it will dissipate its efforts, and will have little impact on any group. In New South Wales, the target population has been clearly defined – they are the seriously mentally ill. No one else will care for them if the public mental health service does not, and without care they will lead an impoverished life, be exploited, cause a heavy burden to their relatives, and be frequently readmitted to hospital. They must be our top priority.

Have clear principles of care

These should be relevant to the chosen target group. Assuming that the seriously mentally ill have been targeted, the following criteria apply.

(a) The service should be easily accessible and have the capacity to respond quickly, 24 hours a day. It should be mobile, so that people can be seen at home if they cannot, or will not come to the service.

(b) It should be intensive in the acute stages of the person's illness. If necessary, quite a long period should be spent with the person and his/her relatives at the initial session, and frequent visiting, even several times a day, is likely to be necessary at the beginning. This is time well spent. It helps to form a relationship between staff, patient, and relatives, and gives the latter the feeling that the service means what it says when it claims to be accessible and responsive.

(c) Patient and relatives should be involved in planning and implementing treatment.

(d) The service should be attentive to the needs of relatives and others in the social network, as well as those of the patient: if relatives are under stress, then this burden should be attended to. Sometimes staff take the patient out in their car while they do other visits. This has the advantage of giving both the patient and the relatives a break from each other, allowing the staff member to assess the patient clinically and, most importantly, allowing the patient and the member of staff to relate to each other as people.

(e) There should be an assertive approach. The service puts an expectation on the patient to behave normally, but it is also concerned to make sure that the patient stays in treatment, and if he/she does not attend for appointments, it goes out to him/her.

(f) There should be continuous care by the one service: it is at the point of transfer of care from one service to another that patients get lost to follow-up. Having one service responsible for a given catchment area – for both hospital and community components – reduces this risk.

(g) Practical help should be given. Seriously mentally ill people often lack basic necessities. The service needs to deal with this lack, to ensure the patient's survival in the community. Staff should not consider it beneath their dignity to help a patient clean up his/her flat.

(h) Care should be on-going. The service must not only attend to the acute phase of a person's illness; it must also make sure that the person stays in care for as long as necessary. Some form of case management or use of a key worker is the best way to make this happen.

(i) There must be a comprehensive range of services; patients need more than just medication and a regular review of symptoms. Some need social activities, others need vocational training, some need special accommodation, and some have family problems which require help. An area mental health service does not have to provide all these, but it should make sure that, as far as possible, some organisation or service is available in the area to meet such needs.

Organise services so that the principles of care can be provided to the target group

In New South Wales, the seriously mentally ill are the target group, and the model shown in Figure 3.3 is the one which is believed to be most likely to give comprehensive care. At the top of the diagram there is the patient, who, it should not be forgotten, is part of a social network. Below the patient is a large box, representing the area mental health service; all the components within the box are services which are provided directly by this mental health service. There is one mental health service for the area, encompassing both hospital and community components, and it is under one leader.

Most patients enter the service via the community mental health centre and its routine assessment service. A number will be in some kind of emergency, and will need more intensive care than a 9 a.m.

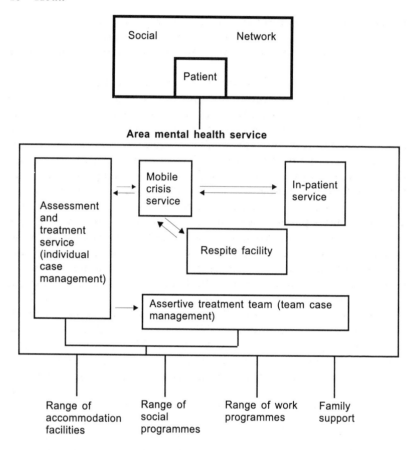

Fig. 3.3. Organisation of the area mental health service

to 5 p.m. service can give; these patients are seen by the mobile, 24-hour crisis service. This service is provided either by a separate crisis team, or by the community staff rostering themselves in such a way that several people are available on a morning and on an evening shift, seven days a week, to deal with any new emergency as well as with emergency cases from previous shifts whose symptoms are now beginning to subside. The crisis service is the gatekeeper to hospital. A patient is not admitted to hospital unless he/she has first been assessed by the crisis service; only if the latter cannot deal with the patient is he/she admitted.

A useful facility to have is a respite house, where people who do not need to be admitted to hospital but who cannot stay with families or in rented accommodation can be temporarily housed. In Sydney, the respite houses are ordinary houses in the suburbs; they are not staffed, but the crisis service must visit their patients in the house twice a day.

Early discharge from hospital is usually possible because the crisis service is able to visit frequently, and to monitor and support the patient and social network. When the acute episode has subsided, the patient is managed by the management staff of the area service. In most cases, this will be individual management, where one of the community mental health centre staff acts as key worker. However, for those patients who are the most difficult to manage – because of medication non-compliance, co-existent drug or alcohol abuse, or family disturbance – a special assertive follow-up team is provided. This team has a patient:staff ratio no greater than 10:1; patients are seen frequently, even daily, to ensure medication compliance and avoidance of conflict, and to try to bring stability to the patients' life. In these instances, case management is by the team, rather than by an individual staff member, so that the load is shared, and the patient has someone familiar to see him/her at times when an individual key worker might not be available. The available evidence shows that such teams are able to bring about stability to the lives of many of these most difficult patients over 6 to 12 months. Throughout the service, the case managers, whether individual or team, are responsible for ensuring that the patients' accommodation, social, occupational, and other needs are met. Such programmes do not have to be provided directly by the area mental health service, but the service should ensure that they are provided, and that it gives adequate liaison and support to these facilities and to the service's patients who are receiving help from them. Psychiatric consultants and registrars follow their patients through the various components of the service, that is they work both in the hospital or the crisis service and in the community mental health centre.

Conclusions

Clinicians can bring about change, but they have to combine with like-minded colleagues, and continue to lobby. Sooner or later, opportunities for change will present themselves and must be grasped. This is not a magical solution; but it is how change comes about. The key ingredient is persistence. Without that, we will never bring about the changes which research has shown can secure improved outcomes for our patients.

References

BRAUN, P., KOCHANSKY, G., SHARPIRO, R., *et al* (1981) Overview: deinstitutionalization of psychiatric patients, a critical review of outcome studies. *American Journal of Psychiatry*, **136**, 736 – 749.

CASS, Y. & LAPSLEY, H. (1983) The costing study. In *Psychiatric Hospital Versus Hospital Versus Community Treatment – A Controlled Study*. Sydney: Department of Health, New South Wales.

HOULT, J. (1986) Community care of the acutely mentally ill. *British Journal of Psychiatry*, **149**, 137 – 144.

KEISLER, C.A. (1982) Mental hospitals and alternative care: non-institutionalisation as potential policy for mental patients. *American Psychologist*, **37**, 349 – 360.

MILLER, A.D. (1985) Deinstitutionalization in retrospect. *Psychiatric Quarterly*, **57**, 106 – 172.

REYNOLDS, I., JONES, J.E., BERRY, D.W., *et al* (1990) A crisis team for the mentally ill: the effect on patients, relatives and admissions. *Medical Journal of Australia*, **152**, 646 – 652.

STEIN, L.I., TEST, M.A. & MARX, A.J. (1975) Alternative to the hospital: a controlled study. *American Journal of Psychiatry*, **132**, 517 – 522.

TEESSON, M. & BUHRICH, N. (1990) Prevalence of schizophrenia in a refuge for homeless men: a five-year follow up. *Psychiatric Bulletin*, **14**, 597 – 600.

4 Developments in Auckland, New Zealand

PETER McGEORGE

In July 1990, the Auckland Area Health Board approved a five-year strategy to develop mental health services in the Auckland region. With the assistance of John Jenkins, who was engaged as a Mental Health Consultant, a costed and scheduled implementation plan was produced, based on this strategy. It has laid the foundation for a dramatic and comprehensive change in the delivery of mental health services in the region.

Demography and social context

Population

Auckland is the largest city in New Zealand, with a regional population of one million people. It is the largest Polynesian city in the world: at least 13% of its population are indigenous Maori and 9% are Pacific Island people. Recently, as a result of deliberate Government policy, the Chinese community has been growing rapidly and now forms 2% of the Auckland population.

Health service organisations

The region is divided into three health districts, each serving approximately 300 000 people and administered by the Auckland Area Health Board through district general managers. However, as described in this chapter, since 1989 the city's mental health services have been managed as an operational unit. At present, the services are being restructured into a purchaser – provider configuration. As part of this process, operational responsibility for mental health services is being devolved to district management.

Economics and social stress

The city has the usual range of affluence and poverty, but the extremes between the rich and the poor have been widening recently, as Government-initiated deflationary pressures have taken effect. New Zealand now has one of the lowest rates of inflation in the Western world, but this has been associated with dramatic increases in unemployment and a reduction of around 12% in disability benefits. This has seriously threatened both the security of people with severe psychiatric disability and the hard-won independence of some individuals and their carers. Auckland compares favourably, in terms of social indicators and stability, with many cities in the Western world. However, there was an alarming three-fold increase in violent offences during 1991.

As the New Zealand Criminal Justice Act allows the direct committal of psychiatrically disordered offenders from Courts to psychiatric hospitals for remand, assessment, or treatment, such a general increase in violence has an impact on the mental health services. Those considered violent as a result of their psychiatric disorder are estimated at around 1% of the users of these services; this is estimated to be at least 100 people, of whom 40 may present an imminent risk to others.

Cultural initiatives

There are important differences between the ways that European and Polynesian people respectively express their psychiatric difficulties. For instance, the percentage of Polynesian people dealt with by the forensic psychiatric services is much greater than would be expected, while the percentage of Europeans who commit suicide is also greater than those of other races. To accommodate the particular needs of Maori people, culturally-specific initiatives have been developed in line with what is regarded as a renaissance of Maori culture. This has involved a focus on land rights, language, and the requirement for Government departments to adjust their policies in accordance with the principles of the Treaty of Waitangi, which established a covenant between the Crown and the Maori people in 1840.

Age-related conditions

The age spectrum varies from district to district in Auckland, but the overall percentage of the elderly in the population is beginning to increase. At the same time, however, adolescent suicide and drug abuse, particularly of solvents, have increased recently, as they have in other Western cultures. All such changes will have an effect on the mental health services.

Social change

New Zealand has undergone rapid and extensive changes in its social policy and economic system over the past seven years, although many people from overseas would still perceive it as being a country which values a simple pastoral life. However, it long ago acquired a reputation for being a laboratory of social change. New Zealand led the world with the establishment of the welfare state in the 1930s and, over recent years, has been an experimental testing ground for a highly deregulated economy. Exports and the gross domestic product are growing, and the country has a positive trade surplus. An increasing sense of competence, openness, and excitement is growing in various sectors of the population, who were previously caught in a culturally sanctioned torpor. Nevertheless, many others are change weary and have suffered considerable hardship.

Clinical context

Beds

Services in psychiatric hospitals were changing throughout the 1950s and 1960s, in line with the advances in psychiatry that were being made elsewhere in the world. Both the use of medication and psychosocial advances in treatment resulted in a decline in bed numbers from nearly 2500 in the 1960s, to less than 1000 in the early 1980s (Fig. 4.1).

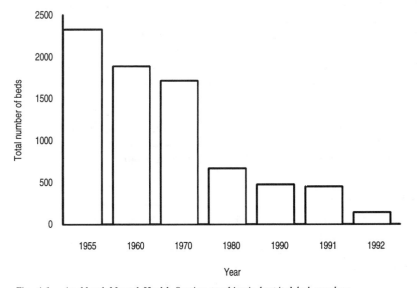

Fig. 4.1. Auckland Mental Health Service: psychiatric hospital bed numbers

Community care and neglect

In 1975, a special grant from the Government enabled the establishment of the first community-based facilities in Auckland. In a move that is easy to question with hindsight, the Auckland Hospital Board established community mental health centres which provided a service for people with minor or moderate disability, rather than supported accommodation or community-based rehabilitation for the longer-term seriously disabled. A split between hospital care and community care was thus created from which it has taken 15 years to recover. Certainly, there were some benefits; for instance, women with depression reactive to stresses associated with their social roles (and resulting in suburban neurosis) were no longer admitted to hospital. However, as in other countries, there was an increased emphasis on people who were considered to be treatable. Family therapies for the moderately disabled became popular, while people with serious psychiatric disabilities were regarded simply as being institutionalised, rather than ill or having specific needs. Their discharge into the community without appropriate support services was therefore justified in terms of normalisation ideology.

This process of change was accompanied by a series of tragic incidents involving deaths in both the hospital and the community, and what could only be described for a time as industrial and clinical anarchy. For example, having prepared for the closure of its secure unit for over a year, with the establishment of new rehabilitation units (both open and closed), the Board abruptly decided overnight to close its secure unit and to change its plans to reaccommodate forensic patients in the new units. The unions with whom negotiations

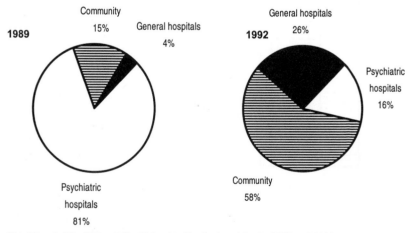

Fig. 4.2.   Aukland Mental Health Service: distribution of funds, 1989 and 1992

had been held to facilitate the change felt betrayed; they therefore resisted management directives for further services changes. As if this were not enough, the Auckland Hospital Board got itself into serious financial difficulties: as a result, it was dismissed and replaced by a Commissioner in 1989.

In spite of a decrease in the number of people in the hospitals, funds were not transferred to the community with the patients and, as late as 1989, well over 80% of the psychiatric budget was still being spent on hospital care, even though less than 5% of the patient caseload was being cared for in hospital. A grotesque misallocation of funding, similar to that referred to by Stephen Dorrell (Chapter 16, p.129), occurred in New Zealand as it had in the UK. However, by 1992, only 42% of the budget was being spent on hospital care (Fig. 4.2).

Precursors of change

Change generally takes place slowly at first and then accelerates rapidly, at times threatening to sweep all before it, and Auckland's experience has been no exception. The first proposal for a system of comprehensive care was made in 1984 by the Auckland Council of Psychiatrists, a group representing both members of the Royal Australian & New Zealand College of Psychiatrists and others working in the Auckland Hospital Board's services. Their proposals were largely ignored. In 1987, a mental health planning group was established by the Board, and the Strategic Plan which it produced was the basis of the firm plan that was produced in 1990.

In 1989, mental health services were established as a regional operational unit, under a Director – myself. The arrival of David King as General Manager of the new Area Health Board spurred the process of development. Working with the Commissioner, Harold Titter, he offered support and advocacy for mental health and, in 1992, Auckland was fortunate to have a new Board, chaired by an adept and determined local politician, Gary Taylor, who was similarly committed to the process of change. An equally fortuitous relationship was struck between John Jenkins and myself, when I visited the UK in 1990. Mr Jenkins was to prove invaluable in assisting the development and implementation of a system of comprehensive care in Auckland.

In 1990, a five-year strategy for change was developed and approved by the Auckland Area Health Board, followed by a costed and scheduled implementation plan based on this strategy. Towards the end of that year, a Government initiative allocating NZ $6.8m (£2.3m) to Auckland for the development of community-based services could not have come at a better time, providing as it did essential bridging finance to kick-start the project.

Components of change

The implementation plan imposed a structure on what had been a somewhat anarchic process: for the first time, patients and their needs were considered in a systematic fashion. Nevertheless, the plan had to be adapted in the light of ongoing events and of responses to the change process. Revisions of the plan were made in 1991, adding in-patient services for people who were not ready for relocation to the community, or who required longer-term care than was appropriate in the new acute wards. Experience has shown the following components of the process of change to be important.

A costed/scheduled plan

As indicated, the situation facing the Auckland Board was extremely challenging, given a context in which ad hoc, crisis-driven changes had taken place over a number of years, associated with simultaneous radical change that had been initiated by the Government and had taken place at a national level. Furthermore, while it was known that the scaling down of psychiatric hospitals and the development of comprehensive local services is an exceedingly complex task, we did not have any first-hand experience. The costed/scheduled plan was an essential starting-point in the change process.

Management structure

A regional structure for mental health that is separate from general health services has been essential for the successful organisation of planning, policy development, industrial relations, finances, and clinical coordination during the process of change. In the move from hospital-based services to local community services, a single unit of management for mental health in Auckland has ensured that developments are kept on track and that provider functions are coordinated, one with another.

Consultation

The bringing together of stakeholders in the process of change is essential. In Auckland, this was undertaken in a number of settings over several months, before the strategic and implementation plans were developed. Stakeholders included clinicians, managers, local government and national politicians, voluntary providers, and service users. Initially, an open-ended process of seeking opinions about existing services was undertaken which included all types of service, for example acute and continuing care adult services, services for the elderly, and those for children and adolescents. The process of consultation was then concentrated on each draft of the plan. Both written and verbal submissions were called for and considered by the Board's mental health service development group: out of 110, only 10 were not supportive of the plan. This consultation process resulted in the plan that was approved by the Board at the end of 1990.

Consultation for change, however, is not without inherent contradictions. For example, non-governmental organisations, while supportive of community care, were not entirely sympathetic to the proposals for professional in-patient care and had to be gently persuaded that beds, particularly secure beds, were essential. On the other hand, many clinicians were not at all accepting of comprehensive community care, quoting liberally from failures cited in the literature. Although all opinions were listened to and were influential in shaping the configuration of the new service, they were not always to be heeded. If all were followed, without discrimination and a sense of strategic purpose, no change would occur at all; certainly no model of comprehensive care could then be developed.

Needs assessment

While a comprehensive assessment of needs would ideally have been undertaken both in the community and in the hospitals, this was unrealistic in the context of considerable political upheaval. Instead, a decision was made to do a general categorisation of patient groups based on those in the existing service, and a more detailed assessment later based on disability, when decisions had been made about where people were to be relocated. Such an approach proved vital because it moved a system, already burdened with ad hoc and crisis-driven change, into action.

Policy development

This was based on the consultative process, existing literature, and solutions that had been worked out to chronic unresolved problems. One of these was a perceived acute bed shortage which had plagued Auckland for several years, despite the potential availability of a considerable number of beds at the two major psychiatric hospitals in Auckland – Carrington and Kingseat.

Services/facilities

Broad service areas were defined as general adult, acute services, rehabilitation and continuing care, elderly, child and adolescent, Maori health, and forensic. Service components were then specified within each of these areas, based on extant models of comprehensive care, consultation, and previous planning.

(a) District-based services (north/west, south, and central) have the following components of service: community mental health centres; rapid response teams (24 hours/7 days a week); continuing care and rehabilitation teams; work skills and drop-in centres; supervised hostels and supported homes; acute in-patient units on general hospital sites for the general adult population and the elderly; and specialised community services for the young and elderly.

(b) Regional services include: forensic psychiatry, psychotherapy, services for people with psychosomatic disorder, and Maori health.

Finances

Based on an allocated budget of NZ $55.8m (£18.6m), staff profiles and operating costs for each of the new services were developed, as well as estimates of the capital requirements for each element of service. It was anticipated that additional funds would be available from Social Welfare benefits and from the New Zealand Housing Corporation, for running supported community accommodation, if houses were purchased by a Trust especially established for the purpose. Such a Trust was therefore set up by the Board. The bridging finance provided by the Government referred to above was also essential during the establishment of new services.

Information systems

A Research & Development Unit was established with the initial task of developing a patient information system; it was anticipated that the Unit would play a role later in evaluating the new services. In addition, outputs were identified for each service and were reported, along with finance, to the general manager on a monthly basis.

Quality assurance

A Quality Assurance Unit was established in 1991. It played a role in setting up quality management processes, with quality being coordinated on a district and regional basis. Complaints and incident-reporting mechanisms were improved and, initially, there was an increase in complaints over the course of 1991. However, in 1992 complaints dropped by 50%.

Training

Given the massive attitudinal and practical shifts required by staff, a Regional Training Unit was established to help their orientation and retraining. It also provides general programmes in which non-government and Board staff alike can participate.

Bicultural

The principles of the Treaty of Waitangi, which is concerned with self-determination on the one hand and partnership on the other, governed the development of Maori Health Units. These aimed to provide care for and by Maori people, and are a result of a blend of Western medicine and traditional healing. In addition, policies of consulting with Maori people on matters affecting them and of increasing the proportion of Maori staff working in the services have led to a greater cultural awareness and to more sensitive services than previously existed.

Progress

Figure 4.3 illustrates the development of services over recent years. It should be noted that minor changes were made to the original plan, based essentially on making greater provision for high-risk patients in in-patient rehabilitation units. In addition, other services were added to the plan to meet the special needs of refugees and of patients with a dual diagnosis of psychiatric disorder and substance abuse.

Summary of progress up until November 1992

(a) All community teams are in place, with the exception of two child and adolescent teams in the central and northern districts, and a psychogeriatric team in the south.

(b) Three new acute in-patient units have been established – two in the north/western district and one in the central health districts. The last, in the south, will be established in 1993.

(c) Two rehabilitation hostels and three supported homes have been established; two more rehabilitation hostels and two supported homes remain to be developed. Also, 56 new medium-stay rehabilitation beds have been completed (Fig. 4.4).

(d) Contracts for 154 beds in supported community accommodation have been awarded to non-governmental organisations (NGOs).

(e) A purpose-built medium secure unit, a forensic transition

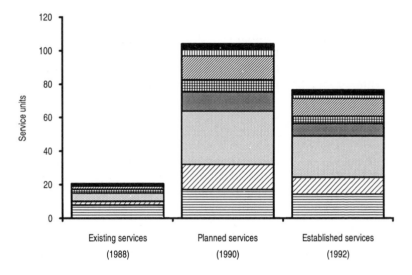

Fig. 4.3.   The development of mental health services in Auckland: planned/established services (⊟general adult;⊘acute;▦rehabilitation and community care;▨psychogeriatric,⊞child and adolescent;▨forensic;⊞Maori health;■psychotherapy)
Service units are equivalent to clinical teams.
General adult services comprise a number of services including Community Mental Health Centres.

hostel, and a court and prison liaison service have been established. This has restored the secure beds previously closed and has added a 'gate keeping' mechanism at the point of previous ad hoc court referral. With the completion of the forensic rehabilitation unit in 1993, an entire forensic service will have been developed, fulfilling the recommendations of the Mason Enquiry (1988).

(f) Two Board-run, community-based rehabilitation centres have been established. In addition, 196 places in NGO operated drop-in centres, and 218 work-skills placements have been funded.

(g) All long-stay psychogeriatric patients (67) from Carrington have been relocated into private hospital care. Two new psychogeriatric assessment and rehabilitation units have been established in general hospitals, and one more remains to be developed in the central district.

(h) Funding of NGO schemes has increased from around NZ $500 000 in 1990 to NZ $2.0m in 1992.

(i) Carrington Hospital (previously 206 beds) was closed in July 1992, while Kingseat Hospital has been reduced from 236 to 140 beds.

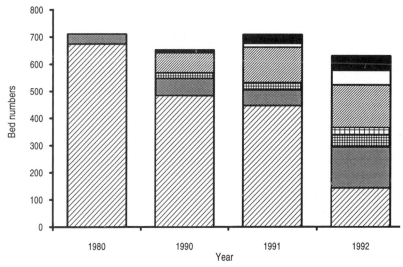

Fig. 4.4. Auckland Mental Health Service: general hospital/community beds (⧄Psychiatric hospital,▓General hospital,▦Rehabilitation hostel,⊞Supported home,▨NGO accommodation,☐In-patient rehabilitation, and▉Forensic services)

Discussion

The experience of Auckland has shown that regardless of how entrenched or distressed an organisational system may be, positive change is possible. In particular, systems of comprehensive mental health care can be developed in the most difficult circumstances. However, sustained vision, personal commitment, political will, and good management which ensures that the right people are in the right place at the right time, are essential if substantive change is to be achieved.

Much remains to be accomplished, including the establishment of respite care, rehabilitation hostels, and services for children and adolescents. In addition, a new acute ward to be provided in the southern district will enable the closure of Kingseat Hospital.

These services have been established so rapidly that clinicians are experiencing difficulty in keeping up with the pace of change. Both clinical coordination between services and case management for individuals require further development, and quality assurance processes need ongoing attention. For some, there is a sense of fatigue with change, in a country that has already undergone considerable innovation. Notwithstanding this, there is for the most part a growing enthusiasm for the changes that have already taken place. Finally, evaluation studies of outcomes for consumers are being established. They will assist with the ongoing process of service planning, and will be one of the means by which a better fit of services to the needs of service users can be achieved.

Addendum

Since the writing of this chapter a further restructuring of the New Zealand health services has taken place with the establishment of a funder – provider split. Commitment to the principles of comprehensive mental health care and the 1990 strategic plan is said to remain; however, few new developments have taken place since June 1992.

Vital time has been lost in the change process. Respite facilities, supervised accommodation, and child and adolescent services in particular require urgent establishment and expansion.

Efforts are being made to keep the original vision alive. Whether this can be achieved depends on many factors including political will, the adequate resourcing of ongoing change, particularly the application of bridging finance, and the capacity of the new commercially-orientated managers to recognise the essential need for both formal and informal collaboration in the development and delivery of mental health services.

5 Self-determination for users in power relationships: the Prato experience

PINO PINI
In collaboration with ALBERTO PARRINI and SIMONETTA GORI SAVELLINI

Health services in Italy are organised into local health units. The Prato Unit, with a population of approximately 220 000 people, is in the Tuscany region. It comprises a number of towns, of which the biggest is Prato with 160 000 inhabitants – the third largest town of the Tuscany region. Its socio-economic structure is based on industry and commerce, and it has strong cultural links with the nearby city of Florence and its metropolitan area. There are six smaller towns (Vaiano, Vernio, Cantagallo, Montemurlo, Poggio a Caiano, and Carmignano), with populations ranging from 5000 to 20 000. The northern part extends up to the Appenine Spur and is rural, with traditional agriculture; the south-west is partly suburban and partly rural, with its major economic activity depending on craft-based industry.

Law 180/833, which was passed in 1978, represented a Copernicus-type leap in the history of psychiatry in Italy, and has given birth to a new epoch. It decreed the eventual closure of psychiatric hospitals, and expressed various fundamental principles, of which ceasing to use the psychiatric hospital as a receptacle for human miseries was one. Another was the need to demedicalise the problems of people in the institutions and to rekindle the personal aspect of suffering at the levels of human relationships, rights, and power.

The Law required that admissions to psychiatric hospitals should be stopped, and therefore necessitated the development of alternative services in the community. For those people already in psychiatric hospitals as long-term patients, the need was to find community services so that there could be a choice. Unfortunately, the general tendency was to re-use the medical and nursing resources along traditional lines in the prestigious general hospitals, so that, in effect, some of the new 'solutions' represented an exaggeration of the medical model. More often than not, staff remained in the hospitals, thus impoverishing the resources available for intervention in the community.

Nevertheless, in the course of a three-year plan, the region of Tuscany has developed services that integrate the hospital and the community, such as a Department of Mental Health. This is a multidisciplinary organisation which has the advantage of more democratic participation than usual by various professional staff, while remaining an all-professional body. However, it risks maintaining a closeness to the institutional model, and of not being adequately open to new community-based alternatives. For this reason, a decision was made in Prato not to concentrate all the resources and personnel in new institutions, but to construct a collaborative network with the other community facilities and resources, from the professional, organisational, planning, and evaluation points of view. Sectorisation and specialist responsibility for a sector represents another important decision which was taken. Our aim is that psychiatric patients should have self-determination, develop new potentialities, and separate from any exclusive relationship with psychiatry.

Evolution of the service

In 1976, one year before the Law was passed, I was working in a day centre in Via Pacini in north-west Florence with users and volunteers. We planned for a time when there would be no mental hospitals; the Via Pacini self-help group developed from this day-centre initiative. This self-help (self-determination or user-empowerment) group involved professionals, users, citizens, and voluntary staff who shared their personal experiences, problems, and solutions as equals. In 1980, this group moved to the Italian Association for Recreation & Culture (ARCI) premises in the Casa della Cultura of Florence. The group had support from visiting other groups in Florence, the USA, and England.

Contacts with France stimulated the idea of providing services on a sectoral basis. At the time, I was working in Florence and became increasingly aware that the ideas and structures required to develop an alternative service were lacking there. In 1989 I decided to join Alberto Parrini in Prato, who was opposing moves toward new forms of institutionalisation of the mental health services. Before the Law 180/833, there were no local services in Prato, they were provided by the San Salvi hospital in Florence. Together, we were to embark on developing a wide-ranging alternative style of service. The users from the Via Pacini self-help group came with me to help set up similar user involvement in Prato.

A national self-help meeting was organised in Prato in November 1989, and this launched the Prato self-determination group, followed by an international self-determination congress in June 1991. Users and representatives from the USA, Great Britain, Finland, Sweden, Austria, Belgium, Holland, and the former German Democratic Republic attended. As a result of this meeting, a National Association of Mental Health Care Users was launched in the spring of 1992. With the cooperation of the Department of Psychology at the University of Florence, a Centre of Documentation & Research on self-help has been developed to examine the effect that self-determination is having on the service provided by the Department of Mental Health in Prato.

As well as self-determination for the users of our service, another important aspect is the development of diversified services by non-statutory organisations, and a movement away from services solely provided by the Department of Mental Health. In Italy, there is a private/social or 'third system', which includes the cooperatives of social solidarity, voluntary organisations, cultural associations, and mutual associations of self-help. The cooperatives of social solidarity were developed in the 1970s, partly in response to the fact that the people had more leisure time. The cooperatives also meet the needs of people who are marginalised (handicapped, mentally ill, alcoholics, drug addicts, elderly, immigrants, prisoners), but whose needs are not normally met by the State.

Our experience is that these cooperatives can be successful in providing a large number of jobs; members of the cooperative and service users jointly participate in its organisation and activities. This helps to overcome the users' marginalisation by the State, and makes it possible for them to become socially integrated. There has been an increasing partnership in developing mental illness services between the public sector and the private/social community organisations, which is an innovation in mental health services. Collaboration occurs in the development of a wide range of projects, including accommodation and rehabilitation. The cooperatives aim to develop projects which will recreate a normal way of life for each person, while the public services support the individual users in these situations.

Organisation of the Service

The current Prato Mental Health Service is based on three principles:

   (a) the Mental Health Service is intended to be a walk-in facility, and it therefore does not restrict access to anyone; there is no selection as to the kind of client who will receive services

(b) clients with all types of mental health problems can be considered by any appropriate section of the service

(c) the principal vehicle for the provision of mental health care is through community teams, out-patient facilities, and half-way facilities. In-patient psychiatric care is only considered as a last resort. In addition, involuntary or compulsory admission is considered by the psychiatric team to represent a failure of their clinical involvement.

In 1979, a psychiatric service for assessment and treatment was established at the Misericordia e Dolce Hospital, together with a network of out-patient clinics. There are two psychiatric units serving the local health service in Prato. The service is divided into two sectors, and each is organised within a psychiatric unit of management.

I am the Chief Psychiatrist of a psychiatric unit which is currently based in an advisory bureau in the town; the sector which it serves includes several areas, one of which is the town centre and four other smaller towns nearby. Home-based care is provided, and out-patient clinics are held throughout the area.

Professor Alberto Parrini is the Chief Psychiatrist of the other psychiatric unit of management. This is based in the Department of Mental Health, and its sector includes several areas in Prato and two smaller towns (Carmignano and Poggio a Caiano).

The Department of Mental Health coordinates the links between various parts of the service – psychology, infant neuropsychiatry, medicine, functional rehabilitation, and social services. This ensures the continuity of all kinds of help for people with psychiatric illness. All the activities of the unit take place in or start from the Centre of Documentation & Research on self-help, which contains out-patient, day hospital, and alcoholism services.

The two units currently provide a service from 7.30 a.m. to 8 p.m., six days a week; the secretariat answers calls for both urgent and non-urgent assistance. Clinics are also held in the surrounding villages on several days a week. There are out-patient clinics at the Centre between 3p.m. and 7p.m. and at Via Goldoni between 7.30 a.m. and 2 p.m. At night, urgent calls are taken by the Servizio Psichiatrico di Diagnosi e Cura (SPDC); this is a small assessment and treatment service with six beds, which is run jointly by the two units and based at the general hospital. The average length of stay in the SPDC is seven days. Sometimes, psychiatric patients are admitted to general medical wards; this has resulted in better integration between the work of psychiatrists, psychologists, and other doctors, and has fostered the development of a liaison mental health service in the hospital wards and casualty department. The two units also provide a service to people in their own homes as well as visiting those who are in accommodation provided by the cooperatives. Table 5.1 shows the activity of the two units in 1991.

TABLE 5.1
Service use in Prato, 1991

	Unit 1	Unit 2
Out-patient attendances		
Medical	2968	1450
Nursing	1170	819
Combined medical and nursing	505	1485
Psychotherapy sessions	821	937
Home visits		
Medical	76	44
Nursing	1326	1475
Combined medical and nursing	249	350
Visits to residences		
Medical	29	
Nursing	617	~~101~~
Combined medical and nursing	831	92

The community services are provided to localities of varying size (5000 to 30 000 people). The services of the units are offered in people's homes and also in health centres, where much of the work is done by general practitioners, community nurses, and social workers. The mental health professionals visit twice a week to give advice.

In July 1990, the Prato service ceased having any dependence on the San Salvi psychiatric hospital in Florence. People in the hospital who had come from Prato were relocated in the Prato area, in a variety of staffed and non-staffed houses, where possible with families. Five people who had previously spent 20 years in hospital now live independently in a group home. We also run two residential houses outside the hospital; clients are admitted to these houses for short periods, for specific rehabilitation programmes. A day centre is about to open near one of these houses, so that they will offer joint rehabilitation programmes. The day service will be provided by six professionals, together with service users and the cooperatives. There is also a respite house in the community with five beds, which is available for use as an alternative to hospital admission.

Other projects and rehabilitation programmes are run by us, in cooperation with the Privato Sociale and other cooperative societies of the social service, currently providing 35 residential places. There is also a self-help project in association with ARCI, whose activities take place on three days a week. An integrated cooperative society is being developed with the aim of finding jobs for mentally ill people;

the first activity will be the reopening of a newsagent inside the general hospital.

The two units of management combined have 14 psychiatrists, 40 nurses, 3 occupational therapists, and 16 psychologists. However, psychiatrists are only 70% and nurses 50% of the recommended levels for staff establishment. This means that the Centre may not be continuously open to the public, even though in theory it should be, and that the rehabilitation programmes often have to be curtailed so that resources are available for emergencies. The two units are also involved in research in a variety of subjects including psychopathology, psychopharmacology, forms of intervention in psychiatry, and the organisation and management of services.

Prato has a reputation for national expertise in the speciality of alcoholism services: it provides detoxification services and investigation of alcohol problems in the medical, geriatric, and neurological wards. Group treatment aimed at gaining insight into the motivation for drinking, and a self-help group of alcoholic patients (including families) who have been helped by the service is also available. It is hoped that this latter service will be extended to other centres. There is also an out-patient advisory service, three days a week, for adolescents (aged 13 – 22 years) who have emotional problems or crises.

The most important development has been that of self-determination for users in the choice and style of services they want. Professionals are forced to seek and try alternatives to traditional psychiatric services and to help the user become autonomous and independent from traditional psychiatric services and practices. Service users themselves are involved in the management of the services which rely on collaboration between professionals, cooperatives, the cultural association, volunteers, users, and families. The project encourages users to develop new relationships that are determined by them and not by professionals, providing real opportunities for them to choose how and where they live.

6 Mental health service reforms in the Czech Republic

JAN PFEIFFER

The former Czechoslovakia has undergone fundamental economic, political and administrative changes. From 1 January 1993 it was divided into two independent republics: the Czech Republic and the Slovakian Republic. It is a time of new and often difficult junctures, but also of opportunities to effect reforms to the mental health services which, under stable circumstances, would perhaps be much more difficult to achieve. This chapter summarises the history of mental health care from post-1918 Czechoslovakia, and illustrates present day reforms to create non-institutional psychiatric services.

Historical overview of the mental health service

The first specialised department for the care of the mentally ill in the region was opened in 1790 in a general hospital in the centre of Prague. In 1840, a specialised clinic was founded under the guidance of Professor Riedl, with a highly developed system of therapy, based on employment, and with a broad scale of work opportunities, ranging from horticulture (in the vineyards) to commerce and librarianship. This became a model not only for other parts of Austria-Hungary, but also elsewhere. The latter years of the 19th century saw the building of ten psychiatric hospitals, with an average of 1000 beds or more each, and five psychiatric hospitals, with an average of 100 beds each, in the vicinity of the large towns in Bohemia and Moravia. They had the character of asylums, but their approach to the care of patients was an active one: there was a farm attached to each (the Prague farm had fields totalling 200 hectares), as well as a number of workshops. However, in the territory of present-day Slovakia, these specialised psychiatric hospitals were a later development (10 psychiatric hospitals, with an average of 200 beds each).

So far as the various specialist approaches are concerned, progress in them was similar to that elsewhere in Western Europe. The founder of psychoanalysis, Sigmund Freud, was born at Freiburg, Moravia (formerly Austria), where a professional psychoanalytical society was formed in 1928. Its further development, however, was first interrupted by the Nazi occupation of the country, and then affected for many years by the communist regime installed in the wake of the 1948 coup.

Psychiatric care under the communist government

The communist coup signalled a breaking of contacts with the outside world and an enforced redirection towards the Soviet Union in all walks of life, psychiatry being no exception. Totalitarian and oligarchical forms of management began to be applied everywhere. Social and economic life was governed not by the needs of ordinary people but by ideological dogma and, with the passing of time, by the demands of the ruling bureaucracy. Among the dogmas which influenced the development of psychiatry were: firstly, a belief that mental illness was the result of bad social conditions, which were a corollary of the capitalist system (under socialism there were to be no mental diseases and no pathological social phenomena such as alcoholism or drug addiction); secondly, there was a rejection of psychoanalytical theory and therapy as decadent manifestations of capitalist individualism – they were thought to ignore the influence of the social system on the individual.

The 1950s saw a reduction in the number of beds in psychiatric hospitals and the reallocation of building use. Thus, the Prague psychiatric hospital became a barracks, its church serving first as a shooting range and later as a store for potatoes. In due course, however, it became evident that the need for psychiatric establishments had not declined with the advent of socialism. On the contrary, the number of psychiatric beds then increased, so that psychiatric hospitals came to cater for double the number of patients they had originally been built for. The biological model of mental illness suited best the communist ideology of the Stalinist era, which was of man as part of the masses; this approach drew strength from the discovery of neuroleptics.

In accordance with the ideology of that time, it was thought to be against human dignity for patients to be exploited through work; in some cases, staff who ran occupational therapy centres were prosecuted and penalised for profiteering and for the pilfering of socialist property. This resulted in the closing down of occupational therapy centres. People were selected for managerial positions not according to their expertise, but for their loyalty to the regime, so that many managers were professionally incompetent. All these factors contributed to a decline in the standard of psychiatric service to the level of custodial care, with heavy reliance on medication.

With the easing of political constraints at the beginning of the 1960s came a gradual renewal of contacts with the democratic world. In 1962, the first day clinic was opened in Prague, and systematic training in group therapy was started. This had a marked family-group quality, more so after the events of 1968 – Alexander Dubček's Prague Spring reforms and their subsequent quashing by Warsaw Pact troops – when it took on the character of near illegality. The situation in the early 1960s had resulted in a ferment of new contacts among a group of like-minded people who had one ideal in mind: to establish forms of care based on human values in a non-institutional atmosphere. A number of new psychotherapeutic establishments were created, psychiatric wards were set up in existing general hospitals, and a system of psychiatric out-patient departments was built up. The Health Ministry issued a number of guidelines, recommending the formation of alternatives to hospital in-patient care. However, the Warsaw Pact invasion of August 1968 proved an unfortunate watershed. A number of psychiatrists and psychologists then left the country for good and, once again, radical management changes were forced through: psychiatry sank back into its pharmacobiological lethargy. Nonetheless, even at this time, a group of people were striving to set up alternatives to institutional care: 1982 saw the establishment of the first day clinic for the long-term treatment of seriously mentally ill patients. The fundamental political changes of November 1989 enabled new freedoms, such as the opportunity to travel and to meet people in other countries. Since then, many holders of leading positions have been replaced, and many new establishments for alternative non-institutional care – such as day clinics – have been set up. No independent group, association, or organisation of that kind was allowed to exist under the previous regime, but after the 'Velvet Revolution' a number of voluntary organisations were founded, including the National Association of Self-Help Clients' Groups and FOKUS – an association for the development of community care. Another newly founded body is the Filia Foundation, which has the task of seeking sources of finance for community mental health projects.

The situation in 1992

Before its separation, Czechoslovakia, with 15 million inhabitants, had 19 735 psychiatric beds in a total of 71 establishments; of these beds,

84% were in 30 psychiatric hospitals and the remaining 16% in 41 wards within general hospitals. Non-hospital care was provided in 239 out-patient clinics. There were a total of 1252 psychiatrists in Czechoslovakia: 45% of them working outside hospitals; and the rest in establishments with beds – of these, 70% were in psychiatric hospitals. On average, there were 35 patients per doctor in psychiatric hospitals, but only 14 patients per doctor in the psychiatric departments of general hospitals. The average length of stay in psychiatric departments of general hospitals was 38 days, compared with 100 days in the psychiatric hospitals.

A better idea of psychiatric care can be obtained by projecting these data onto the average number of inhabitants of a basic local government unit, that is, a town of 100 000 people. There would be on average 47 staff members of psychiatric services: 8 would be psychiatrists and 4 psychologists with half of each working outside the hospitals and the other half within them; the remaining 35 would be nurses – only 6 would work at out-patient clinics, and 29 on wards.

Such a locality would have 131 psychiatric beds – 111 in psychiatric hospitals and 20 in special departments at general hospitals – to cater for an average of 492 cases per year (41 per month), of which 29% would be psychoses (12 cases per month). Of all in-patient episodes, 71% would take place in psychiatric hospitals, and 29% in general hospital special wards. Sixty per cent of hospital admissions would be repeat treatments – 45% of all in-patient cases of psychosis being at least the fifth occurrence during the patient's lifetime. At the out-patient departments, psychiatrists would carry out 23 448 consultations per year, having on average 20 minutes to spend per patient. New patient contacts would account for only 15% of the total number of consultations in a 100 000-strong community. The new out-patients per year would approximately consist of 1000 cases of neurosis (28% of the 3510 new contacts), 560 psychoses (16%), and 560 cases (16%) of dependence on drugs or alcohol. (The remaining 40% of new contacts would be referred for assessment/recommendation, for example by general practitioners.)

In this average community, an out-patient psychiatrist would spend an average of 18% of his time visiting patients in their homes; however, only 2% of all examinations would take place at the patient's home, 98% being at the out-patient clinics. Of the 100 000 inhabitants, 13 would commit suicide in a year, and 27 would attempt it. Two hundred and fifty inhabitants would receive a disability pension on the grounds of mental illness; and of these, only one in eight would return to work, while seven out of eight would die at an average age of 40 years. Since 1990, there was a sharp increase in the number of unemployed psychiatric patients, but exact figures were unavailable.

To complete the picture of psychiatric care, a census at the Prague psychiatric hospital produced a total of 1252 in-patients: this figure represented occupancy of 74% of the available beds; 499 patients (40%) had been in hospital for more than a year, the longest duration being 45 years.

Psychiatric hospitals in the country are, on the whole, in a bad state of repair, and a major part of the care they provide is still of the custodial/pharmacological type. There is little cooperation between them and out-patient psychiatrists. The picture that emerges is one of the provision of conventional psychiatric care at the out-patient clinics, with few non-institutional day-care centres so far. Perhaps the best situation exists in Prague, with its one-and-a-half million inhabitants. Here, there are 2100 psychiatric beds in six hospitals, three departments for emergency treatment comprising ten beds each, but only one non-institutional establishment with three day-care clinics, of which two run programmes for patients under long-term therapy. Prague has a total of 12 occupational therapy centres, each with roughly ten clients, and at least four clients' self-help clubs.

FOKUS

The FOKUS Association for the development of community care came into being shortly after the recent political changes in Czechoslovakia. It is the fruit of efforts by a group of Prague enthusiasts, working in mental health care and striving to create non-institutional psychiatric services especially for the seriously mentally ill who need long-term support. Since existing medical structures made radical changes difficult to achieve – both by virtue of bureaucracy and through adherence to well tried routines – it was decided to pursue the goal of reforming psychiatric practice by founding an association that would be able to formulate its own programme independently.

The structure of FOKUS

Membership of FOKUS is open to anyone wishing to participate actively in promoting community psychiatric care in the Czech Republic. This may include the users of such care, their relatives, mental health professionals, and so on. Decisions are made at the General Meeting of all members which takes place, on average, twice a year: it decides on the plan of activities and elects the Chairman of the Association.

The professional side of the Association's activities is undertaken by a staff of 40, consisting of three teams – a management team, a public relations team, and a team dedicated to the actual work with clients.

The individual establishments (such as the workshops, social centres, etc.) are relatively free to organise themselves. Professional matters relating to the Association's activities and to supervising the care of clients are the responsibility of a 15-strong board of experts, drawn from a wide range of psychiatric establishments. They help to evaluate projects and offer expert advice on the practical work of FOKUS. This ensures a broad view of the problems of psychiatric care, as well as furthering cooperation with important psychiatric contacts in Prague (the psychiatric hospitals, the psychiatrists working at out-patients clinics, and so on).

The financing of FOKUS

The main source of the Association's funds in 1991 was a Ministry of Health grant totalling 9 million crowns (£180 000), but further funds were received from the Prague City Council and from some other local government bodies. FOKUS is hoping for a continuation of the Ministry grant, and it is also hoped that part of the necessary finance will be provided by the newly emerging health insurance organisation and by the employment bureaux. Local government bodies may perhaps contribute more than hitherto. When discussing money, the Association's basic argument is that it is providing a service to the citizens – a service that the state or local government should be providing themselves.

The former socialist economy had at best only a hazy idea of what any service was costing, and it is still difficult to ascertain the cost of health services. This makes it difficult to argue the cost-effectiveness of non-institutional psychiatry. But from the Association's own survey of a 1700-bed psychiatric hospital, it appears that the basic running costs of such an establishment, even if all its staff were to be dismissed and all its patients discharged, would be 40% of its budget.

The activities of FOKUS

FOKUS sets up all kinds of establishments which are necessary for its clients to achieve the best possible adaptation to normal living conditions. Alternatives to psychiatric hospital admission include: day clinics, home care, emergency action teams, various types of sheltered accommodation, occupational therapy centres, and social day centres.

The regional community care model

It is the Association's ambition to establish a model for district community care, and it is collaborating with two of Prague's boroughs (one having 100 000 inhabitants, the other 200 000) to work out a system of such care. In both boroughs, cooperation has begun with the psychiatrists in local out-patient departments, who are gradually being brought into the work of the FOKUS teams. The Association is setting up its own psychiatric establishments in various parts of Prague, and also outside the city wherever suitable inexpensive premises become available.

Lobbying

The task of the Association's lobbyists is to assist in the drawing up of government legislation, with the aim of promoting non-institutional psychiatric care and ensuring the funding of the relevant psychiatric establishments. The FOKUS public relations team has been building up a network of contacts among Members of Parliament (MPs) and with the government ministries.

Professional activities

The Association organises conferences, seminars, and so on, all centred around community mental health issues. Members of the professional team give lectures on the principles of community care at psychiatric establishments all over the country; in 1991, these totalled 200 hours of lecturing. An important part is played in this type of activity by some of the clients themselves, who give talks about their experiences both in traditional psychiatric establishments and in places whose practice is based on the principles of community mental health.

Training

Experience has taught the Association that relatively few medium-grade staff from institutional psychiatric establishments are able to function adequately in conditions of community psychiatric care. Some take a long time to lose their hierarchical attitude to patients, so that it is often easier to recruit lay staff and put them through systematic training. So far, FOKUS has run such training for its own members only, while relevant educational programmes are in preparation by various government ministries. The goal of such programmes must be to help future specialist professionals to understand the needs of clients and to learn to use human relationships as a therapeutic tool. An important ingredient of such training is spending at least a week in the country, in close contact with the clients for 24 hours every day. FOKUS has also been training medical students in social psychiatry at its centres.

FOKUS's therapy and rehabilitation work

The basic rules of FOKUS's client work are: an individual approach; planning the therapeutic and rehabilitation programme jointly with the patient; supervision of the therapists; teamwork among all the Association's specialists; and case management.

Since the Association's premises are scattered all over Prague, its specialists are not in charge of any clearly defined locality, nor do they look after a clearly defined group of clients. At the moment, the Association has approximately 600 clients with long-term problems, 80% of them with psychotic disorder. It provides a complete service, including out-patient care.

The Association receives clients from hospitals and out-patient departments, as well as those who walk in of their own volition. However, since a large majority of patients prefer the Association's services to those of traditional psychiatric establishments, FOKUS is unable to cater for all new arrivals. The client's first contact is with a psychiatrist and a social worker, who decide jointly with the patient on further steps to be taken.

The FOKUS establishments

The day clinic

This has seven staff who provide programmes of alternative hospitalisation, short-term care for acute psychoses, programmes for people with long-term illnesses, preparation of long-stay hospital patients for release into normal life, and so on. The day clinic carries out both individual and group therapy, and teaches practical skills, as well as social skills and communication; it also works with the patients' families. The clinic's psychiatrists prescribe medication, always guided by the principle of active cooperation on the part of the patient. It also provides emergency help, and works closely with a similar clinic on the other side of Prague, whose director is a member of FOKUS's board of experts.

Occupational therapy workshops

These number ten in all, catering for 100 clients. There are two therapists in charge of each workshop – usually a man and a woman. A family atmosphere is an important aspect of the workshop's environment, emphasis being laid on fostering adaptive social behaviour, dealing with stressful situations, and learning practical skills. The workshops vary in the skills they teach, for example gardening, cooking, printing, art, tailoring, and dressmaking. After a trial period lasting a month, patients are taken on as employees of the Association for approximately one year; they receive wages and most of them also receive their disability pension. In the meantime, the social worker endeavours to place each patient in a job for about three months, during which time he/she will continue to be paid out of the Association's funds. Following that, the patients look for a job by themselves, but the rate of successful return to normal working life has been low. However, our experience has been short – one year so far.

Social centres

There are only two social centres offering a structured daily programme for those clients who are getting ready to join the occupational therapy workshops, or for those whose occupational rehabilitation has failed. The centres have programmes for the disabled who are unable to work, and for patients unable to benefit from the work of the day clinic. The centres' premises serve also as meeting places for the patients' self-help clubs.

Sheltered accommodation

This is being prepared: there will be one flat housing seven people; and three flats with supervision from a visiting staff member are to be opened in the course of 1993. One sheltered housing unit will include beds for emergency cases.

During the short period of its existence, the FOKUS Association has been widely acclaimed, and it has received a Ministry of Health prize. It is visited almost daily by many distinguished specialists. We in the Association think that example is the best way to motivate not only members of the profession, but also their patients to be ready to alter their views of psychiatric care. We regard such an example as the essential prerequisite for the ever wider adoption of the principles of community care.

Conclusions

The Czech Republic is undergoing change in the system of financing its health care, for which new laws and requisitions are being passed. This Republic must learn from the mistakes that have been made in other countries during the process of reform of psychiatric care, and it must seek cooperation among all those who are open to bringing change to its system. In short, it must formulate a sensible policy for mental health care and a strategy for its implementation.

7 The development of a local service in Birmingham

CHRISTINE DEAN

South Birmingham Health Authority serves a population of 425 000 (1981 census). For the provision of adult psychiatric services (there are separate psychogeriatric services), it is divided into 11 sectors, each comprising one or two electoral wards. The inner-city sectors are smaller (20 000 – 30 000) than those outside the city centre (40 000 – 50 000) because of the larger workload, which is due to the high prevalence of psychiatric illness in deprived inner-city wards. Four sectors have a mental health resource centre and smaller satellite centres are in the process of being established in five other sectors. I will describe the development of a service in one of these sectors – the inner-city electoral ward of Sparkbrook – which was designed to meet the needs of that particular population.

Before I started work in Birmingham in May 1987 there had been a successful bid for mental health development money, from the Department of Health and Social Security (DHSS), to provide both capital and revenue for social services and health services staff over three years. With that money, we aimed to set up a locally based, easily accessible service that was sensitive and appropriate to the needs of the local population. In addition, we wanted to provide a comprehensive, supportive, and caring service to people with mental health problems, specifically targeting those with long-term illness. Our aim was to provide a service which would reduce stigma and empower users of the centre to make decisions about their own lives. From the outset, Gill Grinham (the social services manager) and I endeavoured to gather as much information as we could about the community and any existing services for people with mental illness.

Sparkbrook has a population of 25 728 (1981 census). Over half the population (50.5%) is from the New Commonwealth or Pakistan (mostly from South Asia), 11% from the Republic of Ireland, and 35% from the UK. The population is mostly in social classes III (manual), IV, or V; only 12% are in social class II or III (non-manual) of the Registrar General's classifications. Unemployment is three times the national average (30% in October 1991). The Jarman score for Sparkbrook electoral ward is + 62 (the range for electoral wards in England and Wales is -62.52 to + 72.95) which puts it in the worst ten of the 9265 wards in England and Wales.

Sparkbrook is compact (474 hectares) and has a combination of high-rise and traditional terraced housing. It is the 'red light' area of Birmingham. Before 1987 the psychiatric service was almost entirely hospital-based, with an average of 100 admissions a year and a mean bed occupancy of 18 beds at the Midland Nerve Hospital, three to four miles away. There was a day hospital on the same site as the in-patient unit, but the out-patient clinics were held at the District General Hospital, also three to four miles away from Sparkbrook. Both hospitals are difficult to get to by public transport from Sparkbrook.

Setting up the service

Before 1987 an Asian language service for Sparkhill and Sparkbrook had been developed in order to meet the specific needs of the Asian population, and we were able to build on this experience. A list of service users who were in long-term contact with the psychiatric services was compiled, in order to examine the extent to which the services at that time met their needs.

Our first setback was that the resource centre, which was to be developed in Sparkbrook from an adapted nursery school owned by social services, was not going to be ready for some time because of delays in the social services planning process. The manager of the resource centre was already appointed in May 1987, and the finance was available for the appointment of other staff; we decided to go ahead and appoint the staff, so I obtained temporary staff from the Sparkbrook area. There are two health centres in Sparkbrook and, after some negotiation, the general practitioners (GPs) agreed that out-patient clinics and community nurse clinics could be held in each. The medical and nurse clinics were arranged at the same time, whenever possible, so that they could consult each other. The GPs began to like having us there, and consulted us informally on a variety of problems. From the outset, a nurse, who speaks Asian languages, came with me to the clinic and, although I took evening classes in Urdu, I have continued to need such help. In my experience it is easier to provide a good service if a professional person speaks the appropriate Asian language, rather than to use an interpreter.

Next to one of the health centres was a community centre, which was used for jumble sales, bingo, and so on, and had a small caféteria. From October 1987 we arranged to rent a large room there (with the use of a kitchen) on three days a week, together with one small office. With these facilities we provided a day service for approximately ten people a day. The office had no telephone, no finance was available for equipment, and there was no budget for the day to day running of the service. There was difficulty about who should pay the rent (£20 a week) – health or social services? Eventually, we did manage to get a telephone installed and another office for the team base, both of which are essential for a local service which aims to be readily available.

Apart from the social services manager and myself, there were 2.5 full-time equivalent (FTE) community psychiatric nurses (CPNs); when the deputy manager, who is a nurse, was appointed in October 1987, we began to provide more treatment for people in their own homes as an alternative to treatment in hospital. The Asian users were especially reluctant to go to hospital because the staff did not speak their language, they could not eat the food, the wards were mixed-sex, and there was no place they could pray. Although we were trying to improve all these aspects of the hospital care, we frequently found that people preferred to be treated in their own home. There was considerable difficulty in getting the nursing managers and general managers to agree to a 24-hour service for people being treated at home, so that for the first year the nurses made unpaid, informal visits to patients at nights and weekends. Eventually, in October 1988, it was agreed that there could be a six-month 'trial' of staff being on call 24-hours a day, and this has been the arrangement ever since. The nurses are also now on duty seven days a week; they pay regular visits on Saturdays and Sundays, as well as on weekdays.

From February 1989, the centre has operated from its permanent base at Main Street. Although we were pleased to be moving to more congenial surroundings, we were concerned that we might lose our good multidisciplinary team spirit. There was a fear that everyone – psychologists, social workers, doctors, occupational therapists, and nurses – might retreat to their own professional territory. In order to overcome this, we decided to retain some generic duties which all members of staff would perform in addition to their specific professional duties; these included helping the service users to cook the midday meal, being available to users in the drop-in area, answering the telephone switchboard when necessary, helping users with practical tasks, or going with them to places such as the supermarket or Post Office.

By September 1988, the average bed occupancy had fallen from 18 to 9 – 10 and, with the introduction of the 24-hour on-call service for home treatment patients, it fell to 5 – 6 and has since remained at this level. One of the other services moved from being a hospital-based to a community-based service, resulting in the closure of an in-patient ward which meant that two nurses and two nursing assistants could be appointed to work specifically with the home treatment service. This closure also provided the revenue for the other health service staff who needed to be paid, once the three-year bridging money from the DHSS ceased. There was a problem in 'ring fencing' the money released from the bed closure and, for a while, it looked as if it would go to another service rather than to Sparkbrook.

The current service

We were able to provide day facilities for approximately 30 people a day in the new resource centre: the services provided are a combination of those which would normally be expected in a day hospital and those in a day centre. There is a drop-in facility with a relaxed atmosphere for people with long-term disability. Users are able to get a free 'bus pass if they attend several days a week, and this enhances their social life as it means they can also visit other people. Users attending the drop-in centre also get a free meal, in recognition of the poor financial state of many of them. They can join in the other more structured activities if they want to, and these include sessions of the usual range of practical and psychotherapeutic activities. On one day a week there is a special Asian womens' group, and two members of staff collect the women in a minibus. The out-patient and nurses' clinics are now held in the resource centre. However, users are also seen as emergencies outside the clinic times, either at their own request or at the request of their GP or other professional. There is a group which is specifically for Caribbean women, while Asian and Caribbean music is played and Asian and Caribbean food is provided at some time each week in the centre.

The current staff of the centre provide all the mental health services to the community, apart from the in-patient services (Table 7.1). The resource centre building is owned and run by social services, who also provide the centre's budget for food, trips, and other items of expenditure. Both social services and health services staff are based at the centre. This has many advantages because it means that there is one point of access to the services, and users can obtain advice about benefits, housing, occupation, and health, all under the same roof. The disadvantage is that the management structure tends to be rather unclear, with health service staff being

TABLE 7.1
Sparkbrook community service staff

	FTE[1]	Staff	Employing authority
Manager	1	Social worker	SS[2]
Deputy manager	1	Charge nurse (also home treatment nurse)	NHS[3]
Occupational therapy	1	Occupational therapist (senior 1)	NHS
	2	Instructors	SS
Psychology	0.6	Psychologist (basic grade)	NHS
	0.4	Psychology technician	NHS
Secretaries	1	Receptionist/ senior clerical officer	SS
	1	Medical secretary	NHS
Nursing	3	Generic CPNs	NHS
	2	Home treatment CPNs	NHS
	2	Nursing auxiliaries	NHS
	1	Community worker	SS
	1.2	For nurse on call	NHS
Social work	2	Social workers	SS
	0.2	Social work assistant	SS
Medical	0.6	Consultant	NHS
	1	Registrar	NHS
Domestic	0.7	Domestic	SS

1. Full-time equivalent.
2. Social services.
3. National Health Service.

responsible to social services staff and vice versa. The pay scales are also different, and this can result in staff members being paid different rates for the same job. All the staff work in the community as well as in the centre, and there is a rota to ensure that at least one person is in the centre (in the drop-in area) at any one time. The out-of-hours rota is provided by the community psychiatric and home treatment nurse; we would have liked other professionals to be involved in this, but have not yet been successful. Five of the current staff speak Asian languages, and we aim to assess patients at their initial presentation in their own first language.

The home treatment service was set up as an alternative to hospital admission for people with acute psychiatric illness which, in a traditional service, would have resulted in an admission to hospital. The service accepts referrals from any source – GP, health visitor, patient, relative, and so on. Urgent referrals are seen by a nurse and a doctor as soon as possible, and certainly on the day of referral;

wherever possible, the patients are assessed initially by at least one member of staff who speaks their language. Thereafter, the staff have a mixed case load, but always the benefit of advice from someone who speaks the appropriate language if this is required. All the staff carry a limited selection of drugs (thioridazine, chlorpromazine, haloperidol, lofepramine, procyclidine, and zuclopenthixol acetate), so that initial treatment can be started immediately if this is required. If the patient is regarded as suitable for 'home treatment' he/she has a full 'work up', as if in hospital, with a full history, written case summary, and physical examination.

During home treatment, the psychiatrist takes clinical responsibility and does the prescribing as if the user were in hospital. The GP may be involved as well and, on these occasions, he/she will write progress notes on the record sheets left in the patient's home. At night the on-call nurse may receive a call to visit a patient and, depending on the situation, the nurse either goes alone, with a back-up nurse (the nurses have an informal second-on-call rota), or with the senior doctor (a senior registrar or consultant) on call for the district.

At this time, any investigations required are organised: the doctor carries a bag with all the necessary instruments: venepuncture equipment and request forms, medication, and a prescription pad. A folder is made up for each home treatment patient containing blank sheets, a physical examination sheet, and a prescription card; this is left in the patient's home. On the cover are instructions about how to 'bleep' the 24-hour on-call home treatment nurse. Any staff member (whatever discipline) records his/her assessment at each visit, and at the end of 'home treatment' all these records are filed in the patient's main records. Initially, patients are visited at least once a day by a doctor and a nurse and, often in the first few days, they require visits several times a day. Medication is dispensed daily where this is necessary for compliance or safety reasons. The nursing assistants sometimes spend several hours at a time in the patient's house, supporting the relatives or allowing them to be out of the house for a while. Sometimes the nurses do practical household or child-care tasks, because of difficulties in getting appropriate services quickly into place. As well as the nurses being on call for out-of-hours emergencies, they sometimes visit people in the evenings, to give either medication or support. Patients are reviewed twice a week in a multidisciplinary meeting, and a decision is made whether to continue patients on home treatment or to discontinue treatment. A decision can be made, at any time, to admit the patient to hospital if home treatment is no longer regarded as appropriate.

On discontinuation of home treatment, all patients have an end-of-treatment plan, and they are followed up at out-patient clinics which are run at the resource centre, or visited on a regular basis at home if they are unable to attend. They and their relatives are asked to contact us immediately if there are any signs of illness relapse. Patients are also offered whatever service they require from the centre – drop-in facility, group activities, social work help, and so on. People who are known to the service, particularly those with serious long-term disability, are visited at home if they fail to turn up for their clinic appointment or for treatment; the reason for non-attendance is often because of a reoccurrence of problems or symptoms.

The centre team provide a service to the night shelter for homeless people which is in Sparkbrook; a nurse and a doctor visit it once a week and provide an informal on-call service to it. There is a community nurse who works with the homeless on a city-wide basis, and she works in collaboration with the centre. The home treatment team also provide a service for people admitted to hospital following a suicide attempt. They (usually a nurse and a doctor) assess the person in hospital and decide whether or not it is necessary to transfer the patient to the psychiatric hospital or to place the patient on home treatment. Quite frequently, they take the person home from the hospital and make sure that he/she is able to cope in the home environment, even if not put on home treatment, or home treatment may be instituted for a few days. With this system and the availability of 24-hour support, few suicidal patients require admission to hospital.

The centre provides a community detoxification service, mainly for alcohol and benzodiazapine addiction. This may mean visiting the person at home, or having him/her visit the centre daily or attend the out-patient clinic, or all of these, depending on the individual situation. A few people are referred to the substance abuse service at All Saints Hospital. There is a regional mother-and-baby service in Birmingham for women who have psychiatric problems following childbirth; this is largely a home-based service and, in the case of Sparkbrook, the resource centre team tend to do most of the home visits because of the potential language problem. A recently opened regional unit allows for admission in the rare instances where treatment at home is not possible for a case of this kind.

There is a social services hostel, which is a district-wide facility for the rehabilitation of people with psychiatric illness, and some people from Sparkbrook use that facility. However, there is no NHS-staffed rehabilitation facility for new long-stay patients, either in the hospital or the community, although one is proposed. This means that two patients who originated from Sparkbrook have been in the acute ward for more than three years, leaving only four of the six acute beds for new admissions.

Sometimes the home treatment team is in a position where they would like an alternative to hospital treatment, but find it inappropriate to treat the person at home because of family tensions or because the person lives alone. An attempt was made to designate one of the social service hostel beds as a crisis bed, but this did not meet with the hostel staff's approval; they felt it would be too disruptive to the other clients. However, there is an adult fostering scheme in Birmingham which is successful, usually for people with long-term disability; ordinary households are vetted by the social services and then supported by them. Usually each household takes one or two people who are accepted as a member of the family. Occasionally, these adult fostering places can be used in an emergency, on a short-term basis. As well as lacking crisis alternatives, there is no financial provision for alternative accommodation, and sometimes the hospital is the only free bed – although in reality it is the most expensive.

The community worker has the sole task of helping the users with employment and training. He/she runs job clubs, trains people for interviews, and supports them initially if they are successful in obtaining a job or getting on a course. He/she runs seminars for employers, to educate them about psychotic disorder, and visits the local places of employment to encourage employers to take on service users. He/she studies job advertisements for those which are only for a few hours a week – these jobs are not popular with people who are not on invalidity benefits because they can obtain a higher income on unemployment benefit – and has been successful at getting people into employment.

There is also a variety of leisure opportunities – day trips in the minibus, football and snooker matches, an evening social club (visiting restaurants, the cinema, etc.),a Sunday club and, one night a week, they have the opportunity to use all the facilities at the local leisure centre. There is a designated forum for organising leisure activities for the district. Some users go on holidays with the staff for weekends, or for a week at home or abroad. There is a music club for people who want to play music. All the staff play a part in these activities – the receptionist, for instance, runs a fashion group for the younger women. The whole team frequently have meals out together or play ten-pin bowling. The centre keeps a diary of all the religious festivals and important national days, and these are celebrated at the centre with appropriate food, music, and decorations. The team, as a whole, and the social worker and assistant, in particular, offer help with benefits and housing, while some team members, usually the nursing auxiliaries and instructors, help with the shopping, the household management, and the budgeting. For those who need it, there are facilities for bathing, shaving, and for doing laundry.

Two carers' groups were established – one for relatives and friends who speak English, and one for those who speak Asian languages. However, the latter was not popular, as the Asian families prefer to be supported at home. The English-speaking group meets monthly. Sometimes the staff (several of whom have had training in family therapy) work with families on a sessional basis either at home or at the centre.

Initially the medical and nursing records for people living in Sparkbrook were kept in the medical records department, but this was inconvenient since large numbers of records were frequently being carried from one location to the other. Over the last two years, however, the records of people attending the centre have been kept in the centre itself, and this works well. It is hoped that the records of the various disciplines may ultimately be in a single set of notes, to improve continuity of care.

There is a process of continuous audit and assessment of consumer satisfaction at Main Street. This was set up by the Principal Psychologist, June Brown; it comprises a semistructured questionnaire, which is administered in the form of an interview by a psychology technician, and the answers recorded verbatim; in addition, there is a self-rating section. The users were consulted about the content of the questionnaire when it was being designed; it is administered every six months to a sample of day, out-patient, and sessional attenders. This survey gives information about what people like about the centre, what activities they find enjoyable and useful, and what they do not like but would like to see improved. Every six months the staff have a planning day, to which some users are invited. The results of the survey are presented at this meeting and, in the light of this information, the services for the next six months are planned. Detailed targets and objectives for the centre are set; these might be as many as 100 and include items such as 'to cook Asian food at the centre at least once a week' and 'a commitment, by the home team, to a rapid response to agencies and individuals'. The psychology technician then does a once-weekly rating, to record whether or not the targets have been met that week, and this information is then collated and reported at the next planning day. In this way, the activities of the centre are kept flexible and responsive to the changing needs of the users.

The service has now been running for five years. During the first three or four years there were hardly any changes in staff, apart from the junior doctors, and this meant that the team learnt to work well together and were able to devise operational policies which could be used in the induction of new members of the team. Several of the staff have now moved on to set up or manage services elsewhere, and I have not been working there clinically since July 1991. Nevertheless, the service has continued to work well, and a similar one has been set up in the neighbouring electoral ward in Sparkhill; this will mean that the two teams will be able to provide support and cover for each other.

Outcome of service

Good Practices in Mental Health evaluated the service, along with five other DHSS schemes (Patmore & Weaver, 1991, 1992). They concluded that the Sparkbrook team (team A in their paper) were successful in their aim of targeting people with serious disability, and also that the users had relationships with several members of staff, and not just one key worker as in many of the other services; the latter was also true of the other two services which provide day activities.

Between October 1987 and September 1988, before the 24-hour on-call service was operational, 38 people were treated by home treatment alone and 54 were admitted; 37 were admitted without being assessed by the home treatment team. People who were assessed at the hospital were significantly more likely to be admitted; 26 of the 43 (60%) who were admitted without a trial of home treatment were assessed at the hospital, compared with 11 (22%) of the 49 who were put on home treatment in the first instance (X^2 = 49.2, d.f.=3, $P<0.001$). As well as the location of assessment being an important determinant of the location of initial treatment, the time of assessment was also important: 18 of the people who were admitted presented out of hours, compared with two who were initially on home treatment (X^2 = 17, d.f.=1, $P<0.001$). These results are reported more fully by Dean & Gadd (1989).

These first-year findings made us realise how important it was to have a 24-hour on-call service, and how important it was for the GPs and other professional staff, both in the hospital and in the community, to know that we would assess people in Sparkbrook in their own homes before deciding to admit them. We circulated the information to the GPs and hospital senior doctors. As a result of this, and the availability of the 24-hour on-call service, 65 out of a total of 99 people were managed at home in the second year of service. Even then, 15 out of the 27 who were admitted initially were admitted without an assessment by the team, while seven were admitted after a trial home treatment. There was still a significant difference between the initial home- and hospital-treated groups, in terms of the location and time of assessment (Dean & Gadd, 1990). A similar proportion of people (64%) were treated with home treatment in the third year, although the actual number requiring home treatment or admission

TABLE 7.2
Number of previous admissions of all patients treated by home treatment or admission

	1987 – 88	1988 – 89	1989 – 90
No previous admissions	26	34	31
1 – 5 previous admissions	46	50	33
6 – 25 previous admissions	20	15	10

had fallen to 74. The staff were beginning to notice that there were fewer crises, and that people who were known to the service were presenting before they developed severe symptoms or problems. They also found that they were rarely being called out for emergencies between 11p.m. and 8a.m. – mainly because they dealt with potential problems during the evening.

The service has become so well known that GPs sometimes refer people to the on-call team out-of-hours. In these instances, the nurse contacts the senior registrar/consultant on call so that they can do a joint assessment to decide whether to admit the person or put him/her on home treatment.

The percentage of people receiving home treatment has stayed fairly stable at 60%, and the number of people requiring home or hospital treatment has remained at around 75 per year. The number of people requiring home treatment or admission over the first three years of the service are shown in Table 7.2. This shows that people who have had a large number of previous admissions (the 'revolving door' patients) are having fewer episodes severe enough to require either home treatment or admission. This finding has encouraged us to provide extra support and immediacy of help to this particularly vulnerable group. Because some people known to the service present now with less severe problems, the team have developed (since 1991) a 'category-2' home treatment service. This means that the staff visit quite frequently for a few days, but do not provide the person with 24-hours' staff availability.

Diagnostic factors do not appear to be important in determining whether people need to be treated in hospital rather than at home. Although the differences in diagnosis between hospital- and home-treated groups are not significant, most patients with depression are successfully treated at home, as are about 50% of patients with mania (65% of these with schizophrenia), and 50% of those with other diagnoses.

The findings from the second year of the service have been consistent with those in the subsequent years. People admitted to hospital are more likely to be living alone, less likely to be married, more likely to be male and (in the case of males) significantly younger than those treated at home, and more likely to have shown violence during the episode than those treated at home, but there is consistently no difference between the groups with respect to self-harm.

The service has been successful in providing a service to South Asian and Afro-Caribbean people; over 50% of the out-patients, 66% of the home-treatment cases, and 59% of the in-patients are of Asian or Afro-Caribbean origin (according to the 1981 census data, 50.5% of the population were from the New Commonwealth or Pakistan).

The service in Sparkbrook has been compared with that in the neighbouring electoral ward of Small Heath (Dean *et al*, 1993), which is served by a different health authority and currently has a traditional, hospital-based service. It has a similar ethnic mix, with 43% of people from the New Commonwealth or Pakistan (1981 census) and similar levels of social deprivation (Jarman score +52.7, compared with +62 in Sparkbrook). This study compared the outcome of people in Sparkbrook who have an acute episode of illness serious enough to result in admission to hospital in a traditional service with those admitted in the Small Heath service. There were 69 people in the Sparkbrook sample and 55 in the Small Heath one; 70 – 80% of relatives or carers were successfully interviewed within a few days of their relative starting treatment, as well as four weeks and 12 months later, using a detailed interview for assessing burden – the Social Behaviour Assessment Schedule (SBAS; Platt *et al*, 1980). This explores both the social performance of the person who is ill, and the distress of the relative about the shortfall in his/her performance in areas to do with children and the relationship with the carer. Distress at one month was found to be less in the relatives of the home-treated (Sparkbrook) group than in the hospital-treated (Small Heath) patients, where the patients were actually in hospital. The carers of Sparkbrook patients were less distressed by the burden, both initially and at one month, than the relatives of those who had been treated in Small Heath. This may be due to the fact that the relatives in the home-treated group had significantly more contact with nursing staff during the first month than those in the hospital-treated group.

More of the carers of Sparkbrook patients were satisfied with the treatment their relatives received than were those of Small Heath patients (43% compared with 23%), and more were satisfied with the help and support they had received (57% compared with 37%). Even one year after the initial episode, 56% of the patients in Sparkbrook were still in current contact with a CPN, compared with 14% in the Small Heath group. The Sparkbrook patients spent significantly less time in hospital in the first year than those from Small Heath (on average 20 days compared with 68 days). There was no difference in outcome in the two groups with respect to symptoms or social functioning.

Conclusions

In spite of this quick response, crisis, and home-treatment service, the ethos of the centre is of a continuity of care, preventive model, rather than one of crisis intervention, which is a small part of the total service. The same group of staff – the team at the resource centre – provide both the service required in a crisis, and ongoing support and counselling when the user is functioning well. This means the level of support can easily be varied, depending on the current needs of the client, rather than the patient being transferred to another team, as would be the case in the services described by Leonard Stein (Chapter 2) or John Hoult (Chapter 3). The team provides all the functions of the crisis team, mobile community treatment team, and adult clinical services team in Madison, but to a small locality instead of to a whole district. The service is popular with relatives and they report less distress than the relatives of people being treated in the more traditional service. This could partly be because the relatives had more face to face contact with nurses during the initial episode and also because a much larger percentage of users were in contact with CPNs at one-year follow-up than in the traditional service. Similar services have been reported in South Southwark (Muijen *et al,* 1992*a*) and Paddington (Merson *et al,* 1992); these teams also report greater satisfaction by patients and by relatives, and decreased bed usage in the community-treated group. The study of Muijen *et al* (1992*b*) also reports a lower direct treatment cost in the community-treated group, but detailed costings are still to come.

It is encouraging that the comprehensive community-based service in Sparkbrook has been successful in reducing the number of severe episodes in 'revolving door' patients. This may be because of a number of factors – open access, home visits for clinic non-attenders, long-term support from the resource centre, and self-referral at the onset of problems because the user knows he/she will not necessarily be admitted to hospital.

While this type of service certainly seems to be feasible and popular in inner-city areas, there are several rural areas which are setting up similar services, and it is important that these be evaluated and reported.

References

DEAN, C. & GADD, E.M. (1989) An inner city home treatment service for acute psychiatric patients. *Psychiatric Bulletin,* **13**, 667 – 669.
—— & ——(1990) Home treatment for acute psychiatric illness. *British Medical Journal,* **301**, 1021 – 1023.

——, PHILLIPS J., GADD, E.M., *et al* (1993) A comprehensive community based service for people with acute severe episodes of illness. *British Medical Journal* (in press).

MERSON, S., TYRER, P., ONYETT, S., *et al* (1992) Early intervention in psychiatric emergencies: a controlled clinical trial. *Lancet*, **339**, 1311 – 1314.

MUIJEN, M., MARKS, I., CONNOLLY, J., *et al* (1992*a*) Home based care and standard hospital care for patients with severe mental illness: a randomised controlled trial. *British Medical Journal*, **304**, 749 – 754.

——, ——, ——, *et al* (1992*b*) The Daily Living Programme. Preliminary comparison of community versus hospital-based treatment for the seriously mentally ill facing emergency admission. *British Journal of Psychiatry*, **160**, 379 – 384.

PATMORE, C. & WEAVER, T. (1991) *Community Mental Health Teams: Lessons for Planners and Managers.* London: Good Practices in Mental Health.

—— & —— (1992) Improving community services for serious mental disorders. *Journal of Mental Health*, **1**, 107 – 115.

PLATT, S., WEYMANN, A., HIRSCH, S., *et al* (1980) The Social Behaviours Assessment Schedule (SBAS). Rationale, contents scoring and reliability of a new interview schedule. *Social Psychiatry*, **15**, 43 – 55.

8 The international user-movement

MARY O'HAGAN

This chapter focuses on the negative aspects of the mental health services, as well as introducing people to the user-movement. Every movement needs to develop an analysis of what is wrong before it is equipped to make better things happen. The user movement's criticisms of the mental health system may seem harsh to some professionals and managers, but it needs to be remembered that these criticisms are the foundation for our contribution to making better services.

Some users in the movement choose not to be actively involved in working with professionals and managers to improve services. Their roles are to create self-help alternatives or to campaign against psychiatric abuse or simply to develop a critique of the mental health system. Other users, including myself, feel our particular experience and analysis can and should influence mainstream services. This has been my focus since I started work with the Centre for Mental Health Services Development in September 1991. There is no doubt that working within the mental health system can be a painful experience for users. Independent user activities, like self-help alternatives or campaigns against abuse, enable us to define our identity and intentions, but when we work within the mental health system this definition can easily be eroded.

Traditionally, virtually all the power and resources in the mental health system have been invested in developing and maintaining professional approaches. In recent years, some of this power and influence has included approaches borrowed from the business world. Mental health professionals and managers are in possession of their respective intellectual traditions, educational institutions, associations, personnel, budgets, and access to people with money and power. This has enabled them to maintain their virtual monopoly on the definition and delivery of good service.

Imagine if users ran university departments devoted to developing the ideas of the user-movement and implementing these ideas in mental health services. Imagine if users had a national organisation as well resourced as the Royal College of Psychiatrists. Imagine if users decided where the money goes and what services to have. The mental health system would be radically different. But unfortunately the resources used to empower users are a small fraction of the resources used to maintain the status quo.

The user contribution to making better services has hardly begun and it will not move far if users continue to lack resources and influence. However, if the user contribution ever does reach fruition it will revolutionise services beyond the present-day imaginations of us all.

The user experience

An old woman and her granddaughter lived by a great ocean. Every day the old woman went fishing. She yelled in awe to the ocean, "Let me take the life out of you with my net". She always returned with fish and cooked them for herself and her granddaughter. One day she gave some of the fish to her granddaughter and said, "Cook these for yourself". The girl wailed, "I can't". The old women replied, "You must find your own power". But the girl did not understand and went to bed hungry. That night the girl awoke from her dreams to a booming voice from the sky: "You have the power of the old woman and the great ocean flowing into the core of you. Now, take meaning from the rawness of life and cook it for yourself without fear."

Eight years ago in a New Zealand psychiatric hospital this story came to me as I was going through one of the most painful, intense, and instructive experiences of my life. At the other end of the corridor, in the course of an ordinary day's work, a young psychiatrist wrote the official version of my mental state in the hospital file:

"Psychotically depressed, misinterpreting at times. Obsessed with need to find meaning in depression. Hearing voices. Thoughts coming in fragments. Rx Chlorpromazine BD + Nocte as appears to be preoccupied with thoughts – hopefully medication will break the chain."

Other examples of user experiences are as follows:

Guadalupe is locked up in a Mexican psychiatric hospital for years. While she is there, an attendant rapes her in her strait-jacket.

Steve is homeless in the USA and wanders from night shelter to night shelter. The hospital which locked him up for 15 years will no longer take him. Instead, he goes to prison.

Laura lives in a board and care home in the USA where she is 'rotting' her life away with no spare money, community support, or meaningful activity.

A young Maori man whose only sickness is the loss of his culture dies alone in a solitary confinement room in New Zealand, from a complication arising from electroconvulsive therapy (ECT).

In Japan, a man is locked up on his family's request and has no legal channel through which he can get himself out of hospital. He is trapped there indefinitely.

Vicki is admitted to hospital in Canada to cure her lesbianism (so she is told).

In the Netherlands, Ingrid is force fed and tied up by her hands and feet in a chair.

Susan is illegally detained in the USA, tied up, beaten, and sexually abused in an expensive, private psychiatric facility.

In England, Brian is horrified that he was kept in a passive role and was not expected to get any better – he later said that he nearly did not.

Patients in an Australian private hospital die through overmedication during deep-sleep therapy.

In all these countries, users are being prescribed neuroleptics, often without informed consent, when they can cause irreversible and disfiguring side-effects. Users can be given ECT against their will and some report severe memory loss. But in medical journals, psychiatrists write that memory loss is not a major side-effect and that these patients have "quite bizarre misconceptions about ECT" (Kerr *et al*, 1982, p.47).

Many users are being condemned to multiple stresses and a lifetime of poverty, inactivity, stigma, homelessness, or substandard housing, isolation, and exploitation.

It is experiences and events, such as the above examples, which generated the birth of the user-movement. Such movements are a response from the disempowered to a situation that has become intolerable to them. The fact that the user-movement exists indicates that the mental health system and wider society have damaged a significant number of users and have failed to meet their needs. Our movement gives us a framework to understand these types of experiences and events, to provide each other with support, and to bring about changes in the services so that these things will not happen in the future.

The scope of the user-movement

Individual users have been standing up for their rights long before the current user-movement began. By 1970, over 200 autobiographies of 'madness' had been published (Peterson,1982) – the earliest one narrated by Margery Kempe in 1436. From 1868, Elizabeth Packard wrote several books and pamphlets challenging her committal, by her husband, into an Illinois asylum. Clifford Beers, American author of "A Mind That Found Itself" and motivated by the terrible conditions in his mental hospital, campaigned for patients' rights after his release.

The survivor movement became active in the West in the early 1970s in an atmosphere that also produced the civil rights movement, the women's movement, antipsychiatry, and anti-racism. These causes are linked by the quest for self-determination. The user-movement has changed in the last 20 or so years; it has grown from a small, unfunded, purist, radical, abolitionist movement to a larger, more diverse and pragmatic movement which focuses on self-help alternatives and reforming the mental health system. But there is not a user-movement everywhere; it tends to exist in countries with Western-style democracies which accommodate liberation politics and the pursuit of individual fulfilment.

However, the user-movement is beginning to appear in some non-Western countries where conditions for users tend to be worse. In Mexico there is a loose, informal network of '*usuarios*' which has been fostered by wealthy, influential women with a social conscience. Although in the West the user-movement could look on close connections with non-users with suspicion, it is difficult to see how the Mexican user-movement could start in any other way. In Mexico, most users have even less access to resources, people in power, or the tools of literacy than in Western countries. The user-movement is also developing in Japan.

Up until recently the user-movement has involved mostly white people – this is changing. In my own country, New Zealand (NZ), the indigenous Maori are over-represented in the psychiatric system, particularly in the in-patient and forensic services, and it is important therefore that they play an important part in the NZ user-movement. The organisation I work for, which is a nationwide information network, employs a Maori user to work on Maori user-concerns. Last September we held our first '*hui*' (conference) on a '*marae*' (Maori meeting place) in Auckland. Many Maori users came to this and were able to articulate their own experiences and issues which are important to them, for the first time in their own setting. Maori users are beginning to form a network and to organise as a separate group, in order to discover what issues are specific to them.

Like the Mexican users, Maori users rely heavily on the support of their *'whanau'* (family) and respected *'kuia'* and *'kaumatua'* (elders). Maori users say that mental health for them means finding their cultural roots again and reuniting with their people, but for white users from a more individualistic tradition, our aim is more likely to be separation from family and carers. This is just one of the contradictions that arise as more ethnic minorities, indigenous people, and non-Western users join the movement. I believe strongly that Western users should live with these contradictions and make room for users from different cultures to blend their particular experiences and needs into the user-movement.

The user-movement, now more than ever, needs to make links across nations and cultures. A group of users at the World Congress for Mental Health in Mexico last year formed the World Federation of Psychiatric Users. At this point in time we are a loose, unfunded network, and over the next two years we will produce newsletters, six times a month, and canvass for members and financial support.

Differing perspectives on madness

Although the mental health system involves a number of professions and models, the psychiatric profession and the medical model dominate; this model is deterministic and often pessimistic. The medical model places a lot of power in the hands of 'experts' whose deterministic and often pessimistic outlook can put users in a passive, disempowered role. Users become 'bundles of need' who have lost competence and, particularly in the mental health system, rationality. The assumption that users have grossly impaired competence and rationality is used to justify paternalistic practices. Under this system it is deemed that people must be restored to competence and rationality for their own future's sake and for the sake of social order, even if it is against the users' wishes and without their consent. Supporters of the medical model in mental health justify involuntary treatment and detention on the grounds that it liberates people from their own pathology. But people in the user-movement have a tendency to doubt or reject the whole idea of pathology in mental health. They are more inclined to talk about 'distress' or 'problems in living' than illness. The user-movement works on, or at least towards, the assumption that mad people have the competence and the right to control their own destinies. This assumption is at the other end of the spectrum from the medical model as it is applied to mental health. Ours is the self-help or empowerment model which is based on the belief that self-help strengthens self-esteem, well-being, and autonomy, unlike traditional medical treatment. Not all users are totally opposed to the medical model; some are just opposed to its dominance.

How do people in the user-movement explain madness, if it is not regarded as an illness? The movement has drawn heavily from antipsychiatry and the social sciences for alternative views on madness that focus on 'nurture' rather than 'nature'. But some in the user-movement have pushed further than this by asking – is madness such a bad thing? Why should not psychiatry and society allow people to be mad if they are not doing any harm and are happy that way? Surely there is meaning in madness – but this is usually denied to people by invasive treatments such as neuroleptics and ECT. Some users believe that if you treat madness with drugs you prolong it because it is not allowed to reach its own, untampered conclusion. Why has psychosis less meaning and credibility than dreams?

In a society which values rationality so highly that it uses it as a yard stick to test sanity, so-called irrational experiences tend to be undervalued. Some users in our movement have discussed the idea of a culture of madness which would place value on madness and which raises the status of being mad.

Activities of the user-movement

The user-movement works on two main fronts – self-help and political action. In self-help we aim to change ourselves; in political action we aim to change the people and the systems that affect our well being.

Self-help

Self-help alternatives are most developed in the USA, although the majority of users there still have no access to them. For various reasons, an important one being lack of funding, users in Great Britain and in other European countries have not developed many self-help alternatives. A self-help alternative can be anything from a support group, a theatre group, a drop-in centre, a housing project, or even a small business. Conventional mental health services provide many of these things too. In self-help it is not so much what you do, but how you do it that makes the difference. The 'how' is really the essence of self-help.

Self-help alternatives have arisen because the conventional services have not delivered what people are looking for. A user from California, USA told me that homeless, 'treatment-resistant' users in her area would not go near the conventional services but were happy to go to the local survivor-run drop-in. Why are self-help alternatives the only place some survivors would go to? What makes them so different from

TABLE 8.1
Contrast between self-help alternatives and traditional mental health services

Self-help alternatives	Traditional mental health services
Grass roots Community groups.	*Bureaucratic* Large organisations, e.g. health authorities.
Self-governing Group makes decisions independent of outside control.	*Remotely governed* Service unit often has decisions imposed from elsewhere in system.
Participatory Members have equal decision-making power and flexible roles.	*Hierarchical* Clients have few decision-making powers and cannot change roles with professionals.
Mutual support Mutual support with peers is the most valued behaviour.	*Clinical judgements* Clinical judgements from experts is the most valued behaviour.
Choice Choice has paramount value so coercion cannot be justified.	*Removal of symptoms* Removal of symptoms has paramount value so coercion can be justified.
Optimism Optimism about peers is high.	*Pessimism* Pessimism about clients is rife.

From O'Hagan (1991).

conventional services? It is important that people understand the difference. I have collated some definitions of self-help and have contrasted them with conventional mental health services (Table 8.1).

Of course, this contrast is just the ideal. As I found on my visits to self-help alternatives, they can easily begin to resemble conventional services – we then call in cooptation. But there are also some excellent self-help alternatives. I have found that if the service is small, radical, not funded by the system, and does not offer a direct service where responsibility is assumed for other users, the chances of avoiding cooptation may be greater. Our movement needs to define its own standards for self-help alternatives that keep them on track with the ideal (Table 8.1). Organisations which promote good services, such as the Centre for Mental Health Services Development, need to put resources behind the promotion of self-help alternatives which are still woefully scarce in Great Britain.

Political action

Political action in the movement has run the spectrum from abolition to reform of the mental health system. Early in the movement's history, especially in the USA, radical users fought for the end of coercive psychiatry and they continue to campaign against compulsory treatment and ECT. Since the 1980s, this focus has broadened to reform and power sharing between users and professionals. I shall now focus on power sharing.

Our movement has a highly ambivalent relationship with the mental health system. Some radical users will have nothing to do with it. 'Community care' which has been heralded as a big improvement in the services by service providers has meant more of the same oppression for some users. But, given that mental health services do exist in an imperfect and stigmatising world, it is important that users have power within the existing services. Power sharing comes in many forms and can occur in diverse situations from a one-to-one clinical setting to an international committee. Every unilateral decision a professional or manager makes, and the process that leads to this decision, has potential for power sharing. When this power-sharing relationship is embarked upon, problems are inevitable.

Some professionals defend their patch and see power sharing with users as a threat, whereas others who claim to share power with users can have an insidious tendency to deny that users are different from them. This denial of difference often means that professionals do not give users credibility unless they think like them and agree with their decisions. On a more practical level, this thinking can mean professionals assume that users should be able to put up with meetings that go on for hours without a break, forgetting that many users smoke or have to catch the 'bus home at a certain time; or they ignore the fact that many users have little money and should be paid for their involvement if they are not salaried.

Another more obvious problem in this new relationship is the mental health professionals' fear of giving up power. Too often people perceive power as a finite and scarce resource which must be guarded like a rare jewel. But surely sharing power adds instruments to the orchestra, or water to the hydro-electric turbine, and creates something better than if it were not shared. Power sharing cannot develop unless users have credibility, skills, information, and resources. Services need to have a commitment to providing these if they are at all serious about power sharing. Once again, organisations like the Centre for Mental Health Services Development need to vigorously promote power sharing throughout its international network. The British have more experience with power sharing than any other country where the movement exists.

Politically, the user-movement still does not have enough influence. One way we can achieve this is through building alliances with either like-minded mental health professionals or other movements. The user-movement in the USA works closely with the homeless movement because tens of thousands of users there are homeless. There is still an unexplored connection between the user-movement and the physical disability movement.

Some political change has been achieved by radical users in the USA. Two or three States have modified some of their laws around compulsory treatment, but there has been a powerful backlash to this from the family movement which the user-movement tends to regard with even more suspicion than the mental health system.

The transformation of the user experience

In conclusion, I would like to return to some of the user experiences which I described at the beginning of this chapter.

> Guadalupe from Mexico, who was raped in hospital, is now part of our movement and has made a video about her horrific experiences.

> Steve, the homeless wanderer in the USA, now works as an advocate at a user-run drop-in centre.

> Laura, who was left in a board-and-care home found a self-help group which transformed her life.

> The young Maori man who died from a complication arising from ECT prompted an inquiry but, more importantly, Maori users and their allies remember him with sadness, anger, and determination.

> The Japanese man who was locked up is now the coordinator for a Japanese mental health consumers association.

> Vicki, the Canadian lesbian, has written a book about her experiences.

> And the story that came to me, of the old woman and her grand-daughter, is a parable of self-help and empowerment that rose up through the ashes of my lost self-hood.

Finally, I want to share with you something a user said to me:

> "To me the truth of a movement is when people who have never heard of each other, from as far away as New Zealand, England, and Canada, are thinking the same thing. Then you know it is true."

References

KERR, R. A., McGRATH, J.J., O'KEARNEY, R.T., *et al* (1982) ECT: misconceptions and attitudes. *Australian and New Zealand Journal of Psychiatry*, **16**, 43 – 49.

O'HAGAN, M. (1991) Stopovers on my way home from Mars: a Winston Churchill Fellowship Report on the Psychiatric Survivor Movement in the USA, Britain and the Netherlands (unpublished).

PETERSON, D. (1982) (ed.) *A Mad People's History of Madness*. Pittsburgh: University of Pittsburgh Press.

9 Identifying the mental health needs of local populations

CHRISTINE DEAN

The aim of a mental health needs assessment is to provide information about the number of people in the defined population requiring services – both specialist and primary care – to assess what their needs are and what services will be required to meet those needs. In order to develop services in this way, it is necessary to divide the population into geographically defined localities or sectors of 50 – 80 000 (Wing, 1992; Patmore & Weaver, 1991). The purchasers and providers of specialist services have first to decide on the level of disorder or disability which is best dealt with by the primary or secondary care services. The annual prevalence of treated mental illness is approximately 250 per 1000, but the specialist services treat only a small proportion of these – 21 per 1000 (Goldberg, 1990). Most specialist services choose to give priority to those with the most severe disability, so that those with less severe disorders mainly have their needs met by the primary care services, in some cases with some supervision and training of primary care professionals by the specialist team. Although self-referral to specialist services would seem a basic right of consumerism, this may result in a flooding of these services with minor illnesses, resulting in waiting lists and a neglect of people with more severe disability.

The first step in assessing needs is to establish from service users what their needs are and to what extent current services meet those needs. However, the way of doing this may vary. In most areas it will involve the establishment of user groups or, where these do not exist already, of user forums, which should be open to all service users and not just to those who belong to a group. Psychological and financial support for service users are essential to this process; some may wish to contribute their views in writing rather than verbally, either by writing comments or by completing questionnaires. For those who cannot speak for themselves or complain, there should be an advocacy scheme.

The type of needs expressed by service users at stakeholder conferences are for 24-hour, 7-days-a-week availability of help, meaningful occupation or employment, friendship, to be recognised and treated as an individual, not to be stigmatised, to have local accessible services, a satisfactory standard of living in terms of money, a home, food, information, availability of respite, safety/security (at times), and transport. As well as eliciting the needs of service users, however, it is important to consult all stakeholders. This may be done as a special event in a locality, with service users, carers, providers (including general practitioners (GPs)), voluntary organisations, purchasers, and any other interested parties invited. This process should result in a vision and philosophy shared by all stakeholders, and must lead to action.

The next aspect of needs assessment is to establish how many people in the population require specialist services and how many require a service to meet the needs identified (e.g. for housing or meaningful occupation). There are a number of ways in which this might be done.

Estimates from studies elsewhere

There are a number of community surveys (Campbell *et al*, 1990; Fryers & Woof, 1989) which give data about the numbers of people in a population diagnosed as suffering from a psychiatric disorder (Table 9.1), and this can be extrapolated to the local population in question. However, this method has disadvantages on a number of counts. Firstly, diagnosis is not a good guide to need for services. Secondly, the numbers from a survey in one area cannot be legitimately extrapolated to another; the prevalence of mental illness may vary as much as five-fold from one locality to another (Table 9.2, Fig. 9.1, Table 9.3, and Harvey *et al* (1992)). This variation correlates well with a number of measures of deprivation, unemployment, the Jarman

TABLE 9.1
The annual prevalence of mental illness in a population

Variable	Annual prevalence per 1000 population
Mental disorders in the community	250 – 315
Mental disorders among general practice attenders	230
Mental disorders recognised by GP	101.5
Mental disorders treated by MI services	20.8
Mental disorder admissions to hospital	3.3

From Goldberg (1990).

TABLE 9.2
Surveys of the prevalence of schizophrenia

Location	Prevalence per 1000 population	No. in a district of 250 000
South Camden[1]	9.8	2450
North Camden[1]	5.9	1475
Salford[2]	3.6	900
1975 White paper[3]	3.3	825
Dumfrieshire[4]	2.38	595
Camberwell[5]	2.0	500

1. From Campbell *et al* (1990).
2. From Fryers & Woof (1989).
3. From Department of Health and Social Security (1975).
4. From McCreadie (1982).
5. From Bebbington *et al* (1981).

Score (Jarman, 1983; this is a composite measure made up of eight variables – single-parent households, over-65s, children under four years, social class V, overcrowding, unemployment, ethnic minorities, and highly mobile people), and the under-65s' standardised mortality ratio (SMR). These data are all readily available by electoral ward and by postcode area. There are not yet enough data from surveys to enable an adjustment to be made to published prevalence figures by means of these deprivation indicators, to accurately predict the prevalence in another population. However, these indictors will allow a judgement about whether the projected prevalence is an under- or overestimate and the areas which are likely to be most in need of services.

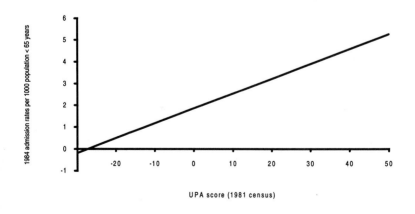

Fig. 9.1. Estimating bed use by Jarman Underpriveliged Area (UPA) scores for districts of the north-west Thames region (From Hirsch, 1989)

TABLE 9.3
*Estimated prevalence of psychiatric morbidity (in women from an Edinburgh community)
according to two alternative diagnostic criteria by marital status, employment status and
social class*

Marital status	Employment status	Social class	ID[1]>5	RDC[2] cases
Single, or married and living with husband	Employed	Middle (*n*=210)	3.3	6.7
		Working (*n*=129)	6.2	10.1
	Not employed	Middle (*n*=70)	7.1	11.4
		Working (*n*=58)	13.8	22.4
Others[3]	Employed	Middle (*n*=38)	10.5	13.2
		Working (*n*=29)	17.2	31.0
	Not employed	Middle (*n*=12)	8.3	25.0
		Working (*n*=20)	40.0	50.0

1. Index of Definition-CATEGO system (Wing *et al*, 1974; Wing & Sturt, 1978).
2. Research Diagnostic Criteria (RDC; Spitzer *et al*, 1978).
3. Includes divorced, widowed, separated, and cohabiting.
From Surtees *et al* (1983).

Estimates from service use

Not all people with serious psychiatric disability are receiving specialist services, so that this method of estimating the number of people in the population in need of services will be an underestimate. About 70% of people with schizophrenia are in contact with specialist services (Table 9.4), but this percentage is less regarding other diagnostic groups.

It can be seen from Table 9.4 that more people with severe illness in need of services will be identified if there is also access to general practice data. People with schizophrenia who are only receiving primary care services may or may not represent unmet need. Another way of assessing unmet need is to establish the number of homeless people in the locality: surveys (Timms & Fry, 1989) find that around 50% of this group have a diagnosable psychotic disorder, and they are

TABLE 9.4
Camden schizophrenia survey

	South Camden (*n*=530)	North Camden (*n*=590)
Point-prevalence (%)	0.98	0.56
	(980 cases/1000 000)	(560 cases/100 000)
In-patient (%)	20	14
Psychiatric services (%)	49	52
Homeless, in hostels (%)	15	—
GP alone (%)	25	23

From Campbell *et al* (1990).

seldom likely to be receiving specialist or even primary care services. Court liaison schemes and prison services can also identify people who have got caught up in the forensic system and who have unmet needs for specialist psychiatric services.

In spite of the limitations of being an underestimate of the number of people requiring services, current service-use data are worth collecting for each locality. The information of this kind required for the needs assessment process is to establish the number of people currently (or if possible an average and maximum number over the last 12 months) using each item of service. For example, how many people are receiving day care, in-patient care, out-patient care, and so on, at any one point in time. These data are not easy to obtain. Health service data are currently collected on the basis of the number of events – number of face-to-face contacts, day attendances, out-patient attendances, and so on – and not on the basis of the numbers of people in receipt of services. It is usually possible to extract the data for admissions, as most health authorities have named patient data for admissions, but not for other items of service provision. A one-day census of all people registered with each item of the service, and those attending on the census day, can be completed with the cooperation of all professionals involved in the service; this would give a one-point-in-time snapshot, and be a reasonable proxy for service usage. A much better method is to have a computerised register of all users in contact with each aspect of the service, preferably including items of service provided by social services and the voluntary sector, as well as the health service. The advantages of this method are, firstly, that it also allows the collection of some information about needs – for example, the number of people with housing difficulties, or the number of unemployed people under 60 years – which will allow the need for housing and daytime occupation to be assessed. This means that a more accurate assessment can be made of the needs of users and the extent to which they are currently being met. Secondly, it allows easy and repeated reappraisal of the users' needs, so that the service can respond flexibly to changing needs or trends.

Survey method

This would involve census or register figures of those currently using the service but, in addition, would include a survey of the homeless, people in hostels and temporary accommodation, and those in prison who originated from the locality. It would also include a survey of those who were designated seriously mentally ill by their GP, who were receiving primary care services alone. The needs of all those people for all elements of the service provided by all agencies would then build up an accurate picture of the numbers of each item of service required (e.g. number of supported houses, number of employment places, number of beds, etc.). Wing (1992) regards a single, basic information system for all providers as essential, because users can use all types of provider services, if necessary on the same day. If more people were to use this method and relate the number of people with various needs to measures of deprivation, it would provide data which would give a better prediction for any new locality.

This method of assessing need and then developing integrated services which meet those needs is a change of emphasis from the current way of providing service, which chooses people to fit the criteria for existing provision. This shift in emphasis was recently pointed out by the Audit Commission (1992). It has the advantage that people who currently do not use the services because they are inappropriate for their needs (e.g. people from certain ethnic backgrounds) will have services developed which are tailored to meet their needs.

It is currently the purchaser's role to assess the needs of the population and to purchase services to meet those needs. Whether this will result in a greater variety of providers and a change in the type of services given remains to be seen. Another concern is the effect that general practice fund-holding might have on service provision and on the targeting of resources on those with the most needs and the greatest disability.

References

Audit Commission (1992) *Community Care: Managing the Cascade of Change.* London: HMSO.

Bebbington, P., Hurry, J., Tennant, C., *et al* (1981) Epidemiology of mental disorders in Camberwell. *Psychological Medicine,* 11, 561 – 579.

Campbell, P.G., Taylor, J., Pantelise, C., *et al* (1990) Studies of schizophrenia in a large mental hospital proposed for closure, and in two halves of an inner London borough served by the hospital. In *International Perspectives in Schizophrenia* (ed. M. Weller), pp. 185 – 220. London: John Libbey.

Department of Health and Social Security (1975) *Better Care for the Mentally Ill.* London: HMSO.

Fryers, T. & Woof, K. (1989) A decade of mental health care in an English urban community: patterns and trends in Salford, 1976 – 87. In *Health Services Planning & Research* (ed. J. K. Wing), pp. 31 – 52. London: Gaskell.

Goldberg, D. (1990) Filters to care – a model. In *Indicators for Mental Health in the Population* (eds R. Jenkins & S. Griffiths), pp. 30 – 37. London: HMSO.

Harvey, C., Pantellis, C., Taylor, J., *et al* (1992) The prevalence of schizophrenia by electoral ward and its relationship to social demographic factors. In *TAPS Seventh Annual Conference.* London: North-East Thames Regional Health Authority.

HIRSCH, S.R. (1989) *Psychiatric Beds & Resources: Factors Influencing Bed Use and Service Planning.* London: Gaskell.

JARMAN, B. (1983) Identification of under-privileged areas. *British Medical Journal,* **286,** 1705 – 1709.

McCREADIE, R. (1982) The Nithsdale Schizophrenia Survey: psychiatric and social handicaps. *British Journal of Psychiatry,* **140,** 582 – 586.

PATMORE, C. & WEAVER, T. (1991) *Community Mental Health Teams: Lessons for Planners & Managers.* London: Good Practices in Mental Health.

SPITZER, R.L., ENDICOTT, J. & ROBINS, E. (1978) Research Diagnostic Criteria: rationale and reliability. *Archives of General Psychiatry,* **35,** 773 – 782.

SURTEES, P.G., DEAN, C., INGHAM, J.G., *et al* (1983) Psychiatric disorders in women from an Edinburgh community: association with demographic factors. *British Journal of Psychiatry,* **142,** 238 – 246.

TIMMS, P.W. & FRY, A.H. (1989) Homelessness and mental illness. *Health Trends,* **21,** 70 – 71.

WING, J.K. (1992) *Epidemiologically-based Mental Health Needs Assessment.* London: HMSO.

____,COOPER, J.E. & SARTORIUS, N. (1974) *The Measurement and Classification of Psychiatric Symptoms.* Cambridge: Cambridge University Press.

____& STURT, E. (1978) *The PSE-ID-CATEGO System: Supplementary Manual.* London: MRC Social Psychiatry Unit.

10 Generating the vision

TONY DAY

Any vision of what services should look like must flow from a clear, basic idea or belief. For Dr Leonard Stein, the founding Medical Director of Dane County's changed community services in Madison, Wisconsin, USA, that core belief is simply put:

> "To help people with serious and persistent mental illness live stable, meaningful lives of decent quality."

That statement generates the major implications that *care must be in the community*: it is difficult to live a life that is *meaningful* in a hospital. The argument is not, however, community versus hospital, for hospital has a part to play. The question is rather one of focus, not locus: where should the focus of care be, not where is it located at a given time? Which is the primary locus of care, and which the appendage – surely the hospital should be a back-up to the community, and not vice versa? It is important to be clear about what both the hospital and the community can contribute to make life meaningful for people with serious and persisting problems.

There is a law of psychiatric perversity: you spend half the time persuading people to go into hospital, and the other half persuading them to come out again. Is that rational? Why do people continue to say that community care is an act of faith, or is unproven? Is that rational?

Care must be continuous. One of the irrationalities about some mental health treatment is its failure to distinguish properly between needs for episodic and for continuous care. Physical medicine recognises that the care regime for a broken leg and that for diabetes are different. When a leg is mended and mobility restored, treatment ends. Diabetes is a life-long condition, and while permanent hospitalisation is unthinkable, continuing medical supervision in the community is essential for some who live with it.

Some services discharge mentally ill patients after an episode, and wait for the next episode and the next admission. In Madison, and in other places where comprehensive community care has been introduced, 24-hour mobile community teams continue to provide support for as long as it is necessary (which may be a lifetime). The aim is to allow clients to lead *stable* lives. In one trial, among people who had been admitted to hospital more than once in the past year, continuing home care reduced readmissions by 80%.

Continuous care of this nature, or assertive outreach, is regarded with some reservation by the user movement. It is seen as intrusive, and there are human rights issues. Some clients have fired the Madison service many times, but they still get a knock on the door, and maybe an invitation to go to baseball. How can service users rid themselves of a service they genuinely do not want?

The service user is the most important person. The key to providing continuous care services of this kind is the relationship between those who deliver them and those who use them. Individual clients in Madison sign their own treatment plan and are encouraged to participate in their own treatment. A continuing relationship with members of a team allows a family-type relationship to develop, and all the needs of each client can be known by the team. Some users at the workshop were uneasy at the pervasiveness of such a model, and raised issues of users' choice.

Services must be comprehensive. People have a wide range of needs, and it should be the job of the community team to see that all of them are met, as well as is possible, in order to ensure *meaningful lives of decent quality*. The Madison team provides services in which the emphasis is on social care; they seek to keep medication levels low. Two apartment blocks have been built, containing some common social areas, which clients of the service may choose to live in. Ninety per cent, however, of the 1500 people in the County who have been identified as having serious mental health problems do not live in specialised housing.

Employers are approached by the team to find jobs for clients. A model is used whereby a staff member learns of an available job and then shows four clients how to do it. They then share the job and the team can give a guarantee to the employer that someone will attend to carry it out each day.

Staff members act as advocates for clients with employers, landlords, and other agencies. They also believe that citizens have an obligation to accept people with serious mental health problems, and to tolerate deviant behaviour if it does not break the law. They work with neighbours and with the wider community to this end.

Priorities must be set. To ensure that scarce resources are used to achieve the vision, it is necessary to accept that they must be targeted on people with serious and persistent mental illness. This inevitably means not developing, and may mean reducing or eliminating, some services provided for people with less serious mental health problems.

People tend to prefer to work with people more like themselves, so why does the Madison team like working with people with serious problems? The team approach that is adopted gives respite to workers, and allows them to share both tragedies and triumphs – you cannot celebrate much alone. The team sees enormous improvements in the lives of some clients over a period of time.

Consensus decision-making is practised and none of the teams are led by a psychiatrist – that is not regarded as an efficient use of expensive medical time. A team that believes it is part of the decision process works harder and cares more; it is not only more democratic, but also more effective.

Despite assertions by clinicians that the public would not support a reduction in popular services (such as psychotherapy), a rational explanation to referrers can help smooth the diversion of resources to more necessary services. In fact, before the changes, the Madison service was viewed as useless by families, by the police, and by County funders; they had little public confidence to lose by making the changes.

Change, says Dr Leonard Stein, is endemic. So let us have a vision so that we can lead change, not be led by it. While some service users find a lot in the Madison model to be wary of – it seems to some to constitute too much care – they would not dispute the need to have a vision.

11 The roles, preparation, and training for professionals in new services

ROGER C. S. MOSS

The main focus for professionals in newly emerging mental health services is that of the team. The mental health system for a given district or locality is likely to be more successful if specific, limited tasks are assigned to particular teams, ensuring that, between them, all the teams give comprehensive coverage for the needs of clients which are accepted by the whole system. Preparation and training for work in a team, especially the type of team which accepts that its agenda is driven by these needs, has distinct differences from traditional professional training.

Teamwork

The basis of the need for teamwork arises from a paradigm shift in mental health services. Traditionally, a caring profession defined its own area of competence, and patients or clients were deemed appropriate insofar as their need could be met by a professional's field of training. If the client's need and professional response did not match, it was as if the professional was saying: "If you do not happen to need what I am trained for, that is the end of my responsibility".

The new paradigm takes its agenda from the client's needs, regardless of whether the individual professional happens to have yet acquired all that he/she needs to respond to that need. By contrast with any single profession, teams bring a wider range of attitudes, skills, and experience to bear on the response that is provided; to a useful degree, the diversity inside the team mirrors the diversity of need contained in the team's task. In addition, staff in teams can cope with more stress than as individuals on their own.

Training for working in a team is more practical and experiential than theoretical; exposure to taking real responsibility within a functioning team is essential. Whatever form the preparation for this role may take, much of the job is learnt, and continues to be learnt in active team settings, so that training strategies will have to reflect this. The relatively narrow specificity of any particular profession's contribution is replaced by a working lifestyle that incorporates a multiplicity of dimensions and challenges.

Although roles and skills have to be discussed and worked on constantly, their ultimate value and success depends a great deal upon whether the team's corporate operation is satisfactory or dysfunctional. A team style that is open, shared, and scrutinised, encourages staff to join in with the enterprise; it supports and encourages them. A properly functioning team cultivates respect for other members' different contributions. It achieves a sense of equality among the persons involved, but does not confuse this with a pseudo-equality which demands that all must do everything, or that certain professional skills are of less value because they are not possessed by all. It acknowledges diversity without power struggles; its members subscribe to a common purpose. One sign of an effective team is that its members frequently share food together.

Vision

Change can be generated by a person of relatively high status, or by managers who decide the course to be taken, or, if possible, by both working together. It is important that a team is *given* (rather than invents) its task, and is then left to work out its way of accomplishing it. The formulation of the task is determined, ultimately from consumers, from governments, from purchasers (including general practitioners), from the justice system, and from managers in consultation with the others. Teams fail to achieve their task when the task is not clear or is too broad, when team members are not committed to the task, and when they do not find ways to overcome their own initial resistance to change.

Attitudes

In addition to a changed approach to working in teams, new mental health services involve a number of other fundamental changes of attitude. These are imparted, not least by role-modelling, team-building, team work, and supervision processes. For example:

> (a) A new form of *socialisation* with users is needed, working alongside people of all kinds, often in community settings.

(b) *Being accessible* when needed, often outside normal working hours, requires a non-office orientation.

(c) The *long-term outcome* for many people with schizophrenia is probably better than was thought, particularly when a pessimistic prognosis is replaced by a belief that people can grow and change over time.

(d) Effective community treatment often requires the balancing of short-term risks against long-term gains. The primary value of *patient safety* has to be re-examined – not all patients who are feeling suicidal need to be admitted.

Team development

Model

As users come to take a higher profile in the planning and delivery of mental health services, it seems appropriate that professionals should look increasingly to an educational model on which to base not only their own training, but also major aspects of their clinical work with users. The emphasis is on learning together, and not merely on the imparting of knowledge and skills in one direction.

Programmes

Team members learn together in a variety of ways, many of which form a natural part of their working life. Opportunities for team training are as follows:

> team building days
> team education meetings – learning a new skill, updates, and so on
> case conferences – considering a difficult client for example
> business meetings
> treatment plan review meetings
> suicide reviews
> client reviews
> daily handover sessions
> interconsultative team supervision – using specialist expertise
> staff support meetings.

Maintaining services

Teamwork is not perfected simply by setting up an enthusiastic, well selected, clearly assigned team. After the 'honeymoon' period, stagnation and regression need to be actively prevented. The ongoing process of the team is part of the strategy for further change, as are experimentation, audit, and training. Frontline clinicians are in a good position to contribute to this with locality-based research. Staff can be seconded periodically to different jobs, to augment their own or the team's resource base. Students on placement are not only learning teamwork *in situ*, but they also have their own useful role in posing questions which the team can take seriously. Good staff-support structures such as debriefing and mutual support groups can play their part in the ongoing educational process.

Clinical supervision, however it is conducted, provides support and quality control, but it also contributes to continuing training. At different levels, it may involve the team manager, the line manager, outside experts, and other members of the team. Forms of clinical supervision include:

> team management – team manager
> caseload management – team manager
> line management – senior fellow-professional
> personal (formal) supervision – selected expert
> informal supervision – almost anybody
> team or peer supervision – team members.

Supervision is conducted on an adult – adult basis as in psychotherapy, rather than on the foreman – worker principle on the shop floor.

Specific skills for community work

The specific skills for community work listed below are not intended to be comprehensive, but to give an idea of skills required by the new mental health services, in contrast with traditional professional training:

> socialisation to work alongside all types of people
> engaging with psychotic people
> conversant with psychotropic medication
> market research
> goal setting and setting priorities
> case management
> social skills training
> use of ordinary settings for clinical work
> incorporation of consumer choice
> networking
> containing a crisis
> acquiring a skill from someone else.

Changing professional roles

In the case of training, as with other aspects of developing new services, the management of change is central; unpicking existing training methods does not need to imply that everything of proven value has to be lost. However, it does require a new look at aims and standards, and this touches on the traditional territory of professional colleges and organisations. The problem is that no single profession would or could lead the way for training across the whole front of new mental health services.

Many discussions of this sort raise the problems that people perceive in their dealings with established psychiatrists. Those who are enthusiastic for new services look for changing attitudes among psychiatrists, and may be disappointed with what they encounter. Psychiatrists are accused of holding on to power and prestige, and of standing in the way of progress. By contrast, psychiatrists themselves may consider that they are looking after the public's interests by assessing the validity of new methods before they adopt them. Not all psychiatrists have to be innovators or active researchers any more than the members of any other group, nor are they all primarily interested in community psychiatry; the profession as a whole has many other concerns to develop.

Solutions lie in involving psychiatrists in discussions about new services from the start; their professional commitment to the needs of service users can be mobilised, not least by the users themselves. Psychiatrists often respond to good demonstrations in the field by their own colleagues. They need to discover the effectiveness of new approaches, and may respond to encouragement to set up pilot projects and investigate them. The Centre for Mental Health Services Development may well be able to delineate new models which professional interests can consider from their own standpoints.

Problems

Some of the relevant issues require further thought. External pressures may have positive or negative effects, for example the requirements of purchasers who may not yet understand the nature of the services, or the voice of users beginning to express themselves more forcefully.

With all the emphasis on teamwork, what about teams that do not want to be teams? Or key-workers who avoid taking key-worker responsibilities? Resistance to new approaches can present as antagonism between the disciplines, especially if team members do not allow the primacy of their own profession's interests to give way to a central focus on the concerns of the team. Not even the team is its own *raison d'être* – the real contenders for the central role are the users and their needs. There is a role for service users in the process of training, and there might be a way for them to have a say in the selection of staff.

Further reading

FACTOR, R.M., STEIN, L.I. & DIAMOND, R.J. (1988) A model community psychiatry curriculum for psychiatric residents. *Community Mental Health Journal,* **24,** 310 – 326.

STEIN, L.I., DIAMOND, R.J. & FACTOR, R.M. (1990) A system approach to the care of persons with schizophrenia. In *Schizophrenia: Vol. 5. Psychological Therapies* (eds M.I. Herz, S.J. Keith & J.P. Docherty), pp. 213 – 246. Amsterdam: Elsevier Science.

12 Sustaining new community mental health services

EDWARD PECK

The range of issues discussed in this chapter can be broadly divided into two main themes: the first relates to the manner in which new services are designed, in the context of the purchaser/provider split and the increasing emphasis on users' involvement; the second relates to the importance of targeting specific groups of users and the issues around the definition of these groups.

Service design

The shape of the service pioneered in New South Wales (NSW) by John Hoult is described in Chapter 3. This innovative service was largely based on his personal frustration with the mental health system of NSW in the mid-1970s. The alternative model was designed and championed by Hoult and, in the course of winning support for his ideas, he recognised the value of:

(a) perseverance – the need for stamina and determination in pursuing the objective

(b) understanding the politics of funding organisations – the need to engage with the realities of power and influence in agencies

(c) starting with a research project – the need to initiate a scheme which would subsequently provide support for expansion/replication

(d) training for attitudinal changes – the need to strike a balance between theoretical learning and practical experience.

Hoult therefore presented the view that the product-champion is central to the creation and sustenance of new community mental health services. This approach stresses the centrality to change of the individual who becomes disenchanted with a situation, decides what should happen, and then manipulates local circumstances to achieve that end.

This view has gained widespread support as both description (explaining how change is achieved) and prescription (recommending how change can be achieved). Hoult's view was therefore accepted by a number of group members, but others did not share this view. They felt that product-champions were liable to be unreflective about the appropriateness of the product that they were championing, which might serve the interests of that individual or their profession rather than address the concerns of any broader constituency, such as service users. They believed the product-champion had few safeguards against the promotion of a poor product and that, in the 15 years since the publication of *Better Services for the Mentally Ill* (Department of Health & Social Security, 1975), few such champions had come forward to implement even these relatively modest reforms. If progress had to wait for champions of appropriate products, then progress might wait a long time. In particular, some members felt that this approach was not relevant to the current UK context in two respects.

The first concerned the increasing recognition that service users had to be central to the design of new mental health services. This is a position with growing currency (Jenkins, 1992), and there was some discussion in the group about methods of achieving user involvement. It was also recognised that there was a need to have an approach to service design which involved users as one set of significant stakeholders in a process which also engaged professionals, carers, voluntary agencies, and so on. One model for achieving a starting point to such an approach, the Search Conference, was described (Wertheimer, 1991); some members felt it crucial that such techniques be established as part of a process which legitimised and acted upon the conclusions of those stakeholders. This might well mean a change in the organisational structure and culture of the statutory agencies involved. Such a thorough approach might well need persistent and determined promotion in a locality by one or two individuals – people which the group termed 'process-champions'.

This line of thought led onto the second aspect of the UK context which possibly made the product-champion theory appear potentially outdated. The purchaser/provider split seemed to offer an ideal opportunity for the development of process-champions in the purchasing organisations. Without a coherent method for gathering the views of users, as well as carers, voluntary agencies, general practitioners, and so on, purchasers appeared to the group to have no basis on which to challenge the products being offered by providers (Barker, 1991). As the holders of the purse strings, process-champions in the purchasing authority had the ability to vest new approaches and structures with genuine power to decide on service changes. This process could involve users in the key purchasing tasks of assessing and prioritising needs and specifying the outcomes that services should meet in relation to those needs, such as what the products should achieve for people. In contrast, the continuation of the notion of product-champions would leave the definition of need and outcomes with professionals in the provider agencies.

Targeting groups

John Hoult was adamant that new mental health services must be absolutely clear about the client group that they intend to deal with, and those they did *not* intend to deal with, and that this focus should be on the long-term users of mental health services with multiple problems. This view accords with a recent review of the literature on successful community models (Scott, 1992). Most members of the group appreciated this unequivocal piece of advice, but with two reservations.

Firstly, members were concerned about the definition of the specified set of users and whether they should be defined by diagnosis or more broadly based need-assessment tools. Preference seemed to be for the latter approach and members made reference to examples (Peck & Smith, 1991) stressing the limitations of diagnostic groups as accurate predictors of need.

Secondly, members were worried about the implication that this set of users should be targeted at the expense of providing 'comprehensive' service to a locality – one of the guiding principles of most UK service plans. Hoult maintained that the provision of such a 'comprehensive' service would typically, in current financial circumstances, mean the neglect of long-term users with multiple problems. There is evidence in the UK to support this view (Murphy, 1991). Nonetheless, some members expressed fears that preventive work in the early stages of distress would be lost, with a negative impact on levels of subsequent need, professional motivation, and skill. Once again, it appeared that this was an issue on which purchasers should focus attention.

References

BARKER, I. (1991) Purchasing for people. *Health Services Management,* October, 212 – 214.

DEPARTMENT OF HEALTH & SOCIAL SECURITY (1975) *Better Services for the Mentally Ill.* Cmnd 6233. London: HMSO.

JENKINS, J. (1992) Failure and the future. In *Community Mental Health Services – Models for the Future* (ed. E. Peck). Newcastle University, HSMU Conference Proceedings. Paper No. 11.

MURPHY, E. (1991) *After the Asylums.* London: Faber & Faber.

PECK, E. & SMITH, H. (1991) *Contracting for Mental Health Services: A Framework for Action.* Bristol: National Health Services Training Authority.

SCOTT, J. (1992) Perspectives on community mental health services. In *Community Mental Health Services – Models for the Future* (ed. E. Peck). Newcastle University, HSMU Conference Proceedings. Paper No. 11.

WERTHEIMER, A. (1991) *A Chance to Speak Out.* London: King's Fund College.

13 Involving service users

PIERS ALLOTT and PAT HOLMES

The history of the user-movement

The activities of Elizabeth Packard and Clifford Beers are historically important to the user-movement as they made the first attempts 'to claim back' what service users had lost, that is the power to control their own lives.

The development of the user-movement, as we know it today, began in the USA in the 1970s at a time when there were the beginnings of awareness about other disempowered groups of people, who included women and black people.

The early movement in the USA focused on a few specific cases and led to the development of radical views and an attempt to abolish psychiatric institutions and replace them with self-help solutions. During the 1980s, this approach developed into two parallel approaches: one with a continuing emphasis on replacing psychiatric institutions with self-help alternatives; and the other setting more achievable goals, with an emphasis on ensuring user involvement in current and developing services. The latter group remains committed to the development of self-help alternatives. A number of alternatives have now been set up in the USA, and other parts of the world, including Holland and New Zealand.

The setting up of the World Federation of Psychiatric Users in Mexico, in August 1991, is an important step in beginning to develop a worldwide network and power base for the users of psychiatric services.

Degrees of user empowerment

The degrees of user empowerment range from neglect and disempowerment to full empowerment (see Fig. 13.1 for a summary).

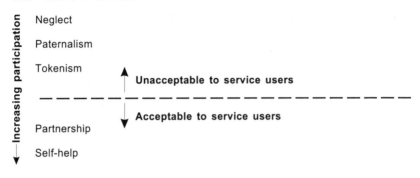

Fig. 13.1. Diagrammatic illustration of the degrees of user participation

Above the line in Figure 13.1 represents neglect (people abandoned in institutions and homeless service users) and paternalism (people setting themselves up to act/make decisions or speak on behalf of service users) as totally unacceptable to people who use psychiatric services. It would surprise most people working in the health service today to hear public admission about the existence of neglect of service users. However, there are many carers, managers, and professionals who would not recognise the paternalism which is evident in the views and attitudes of many. Often articulate service users who have spent years in psychiatric hospitals and who have been defined as 'long-term chronic cases' are openly challenged in public fora about their being 'lucky', but not the people normally seen in psychiatric hospitals!

Empowering service users requires altering the balance of power. This means that those who are in power positions must share power. Rehabilitation of managers and professionals cannot be achieved in one step and, while 'tokenism' is unacceptable to service users, it can be a positive step if there is commitment to forward development. Tokenism may be the beginning of recognition that there is an issue – but it is only the first step towards a more democratic system of mental health care. Within tokenism there may be increasing levels of awareness and development of understanding about the value of user – professional dialogue, and through this the beginnings of real partnership.

The achievement of partnership may lead to a willingness of professionals and carers to facilitate and enable the movement to go forward to 'self-help' (below the line in Fig.13.1) and user-controlled alternatives. This will begin really to test the distance travelled from paternalism and neglect.

Barriers to participation and bridges to involvement

Enthusiasm for involving service users is easily expressed, but it is much more difficult to develop effective involvement across services at different levels and within different structures. The first important step must be the development of people's awareness that the empowerment of service users is worthwhile. Any involvement in planning should be from the outset, rather than at a later stage. Accessible, comprehensible information must be available to service users if they are to participate in planning and in decisions about their own treatment. Resources will be required for user involvement and user groups – for training, conference attendances, payment of users for work, funding for travel, and so on.

Service users should have involvement at all levels of organisation where partnerships can be developed with professionals and managers. At its simplest level, all individuals who use the psychiatric service must be involved in their own treatment. Traditional psychiatric services can be seen by some as invalidating the individuals they are supposed to be assisting. It is important to 'revalue' such people by enabling them to work with others, for example clinicians, on the development of a care plan or in decisions about everyday life.

Action should be general and daily, for example ensuring that user concerns are included at the top of all agenda. Both carers and service users should be involved, but not usually together. It is inappropriate to consult a carer on a user's behalf or to see the voluntary sector as the voice of the user. There is also a danger in asking voluntary organisations to identify 'appropriate' service users. Users need to decide for themselves that they want to be involved and to form groups. One user representing all others (tokenism) should be avoided wherever possible, but it does represent a starting point. The individual user should be nominated by other users and have a reference group. Users need to have a wide network and collective voice to influence policy development and services. Involvement is thus needed at all levels to empower people. Users can be supported on themes, for example electroconvulsive therapy, by interaction with others on a wide basis. It is generally easier for people to advise on existing services than on future developments because they may be unaware of the possibilities.

Conclusions

Involving service users and developing partnerships is essential to the development of effective, caring, and meaningful mental health services. The required actions to achieve involvement are easy. Changing the attitudes remaining after years of traditional training (much of which is current today), and paternalistic systems of care, provide the real challenge to managers and professionals. Service users are ready to begin real involvement in changing mental health services; they only need the commitment to change to more democratic forms of care from those in positions of power.

Further reading

BARKER, I. & PECK, E. (1987) *Power in Strange Places: User Empowerment in Mental Health Services.* London: Good Practices in Mental Health.

BEEFORTH, M., CONLAN, E., FIELD, V., *et al* (1990) *Whose Service is it Anyway? Users' Views on Coordinating Community Care.* London: Research and Development in Psychiatry.

CAMPBELL, P. (1992) A survivor's view of community psychiatry. *Journal of Mental Health,* 1, 117–122.

CHAMBERLIN, J. (1988) *On our Own: Patient-Controlled Alternatives to the Mental Health System.* London: MIND.

GOOD PRACTICES FOR MENTAL HEALTH AND CAMDEN CONSORTIUM (1988) *Treated Well? A Code of Practice for Psychiatric Hospitals.* London: Good Practices in Mental Health.

14 The role of carers

PADDY COONEY

Who are the carers?

The term 'informal carers' is used for family and friends to distinguish them from professionals. Some professionals refer to themselves as 'carers', but this is not acceptable to family and friends; professionals may care but they are not carers. The term 'informal' should not imply that carers have a choice to care – usually they do not. As well as doing the work with people with mental illness, carers also campaign for them.

Do carers have rights?

Carers have a right to be involved in the planning of mental illness services at all levels and in all parts of the process. This may mean adapting the process so that carers can contribute – by changing the times, locations, and style of meetings to suit them. Carers can contribute on an equal footing in the planning team as individuals; an individual is not representative of all carers, but this is true of the other members of the planning team – they are not representative of their professional group either. They have the right not to care without being made to feel guilty. They have a right to some meaningful income for the work they do, rather than merely to receive social services benefits which are felt to be demeaning.

The needs of carers

The perspective of the carer and user are different, and this may result in conflict. Although users and carers are inextricably linked, their individual views should be heard. Support for carers is important, either in a group or by experienced carers talking to new ones. It is also important for them to have ready access to support. Carers need information which is free of jargon; they need to be listened to and have their views respected and to have active involvement in care plans and care programming. Will it be possible for carers to be the care managers and if so, would this be desirable?

The power of carers

Carers do not always realise their own political strength and that they and the users may be more able than professionals to influence politicians. Carers need to understand the role of local authority members and need help in making links with the political process.

Carers do not want to be consulted by professionals when an individual care plan or a plan for services is complete, but to be involved in both processes when there is a blank sheet of paper.

Further reading

HAFFENSEN, S. (1989) *Working Together*. London: Carers' National Association.

HER MAJESTY'S STATIONARY OFFICE (HMSO) (1991) *Getting it Right for Carers, Setting up Services for Carers*. London: HMSO.

HOUSE OF COMMONS SOCIAL SERVICES COMMITTEE (1990) *Community Care: Carers*. London: HMSO.

KUIPERS, L. & BEBBINGTON, B. (1987) *Living with Mental Illness – A Book for Friends and Relatives*. London: Souvenir Press.

SEEMAN, M. V., LILTMANN, S. K., PLUMMER, E., *et al* (1982) *Living and Working with Schizophrenia - Information and Support for Patients and their Families, Friends, Employers, and Teachers*. Milton Keynes: Open University Press.

15 Measuring outcomes

CHRISTINE DEAN and ANN FOSTER

Ideally, measures of outcomes should not be service measures, but desirable outcomes for users and carers which can be broken down into measurable indicators. Currently, most measures are unhelpful, for example completed consultant episodes, number of patient contacts, and average length of stay in hospital. The significance of data in terms of the measurement of the success of a service is unclear, and they have been adopted as indicators mainly because current information systems enable the collection of such data. The current data collection systems to fulfil Körner requirements collect contact data, but not named individual data; this means that it is not possible to ascertain how many people are using a particular service, and therefore impossible to ascertain whether people using the service are benefiting from it. There is an urgent need to develop information systems which record information about the needs of individuals and targets for them, and the extent to which the services meet those needs and targets.

It is essential that service users and carers are involved in the assessment of individual needs, and that they are also involved in the evaluation of the success of service interventions. There should be qualitative as well as quantitative measures. They should include measures of user and carer satisfaction, and measures of users' and carers' physical and mental health, quality of life, and social functioning.

The operational tool which might be used as the measurement of success is the individual client care plan; success would therefore be measured in relation to the extent to which the goals in the individual care plan had been realised. The goals to be achieved and the means of assessing the attainment of the targets must be agreed between user and provider. As well as the measurement of the extent to which individual targets are met in a manner acceptable to the recipient, the cost-effectiveness with which these targets have been met should also be assessed.

Rachel Jenkins (Department of Health) said that it is possible to measure outcomes reliably in terms of symptoms, but these are often lengthy; a short, structured scheme is needed which can be used by clinicians at regular intervals. There is also a need to develop a short quality-of-life measure which can be repeated routinely. Some measures currently available which could be used routinely are listed below.

Possible measures of outcome for service users with long-term mental illness

Symptoms

Krawiecka Scale
KRAWIECKA, M., GOLDBERG, D.P. & VAUGHAN, M. (1977) A standardised psychiatric assessment scale for rating chronic psychotic patients. *Acta Psychiatrica Scandinavica,* **55**, 299 – 308.

Schizophrenia Change Scale
MONTGOMERY, S.A., TAYLOR, P. & MONTGOMERY, D. (1978) Development of a schizophrenia scale sensitive to change. *Neuropharmacology,* **17**, 1061 – 1063.

Brief Psychiatric Rating Scale (BPRS)
OVERALL, J.E. & GORHAM, D.R. (1962) The Brief Psychiatric Rating Scale. *Psychological Reports,* **10**, 799 – 812.

Global Assessment of Functioning Scale
ENDICOTT, J., SPITZER, R., FLEISS, J., *et al* (1976) The Global Assessment Scale. *Archives of General Psychiatry,* **33**, 766 – 771.

Social functioning

Social Behaviour Schedule (SBS)
WYKES, T. & STURT, E. (1986) The measurement of social behaviour in psychiatric patients: an assessment of the reliability and validity of the SBS. *British Journal of Psychiatry,* **148**, 1 – 11.

Social Behaviour Assessment Schedule (SBAS)
PLATT, S., WEYMANN, A. & HIRSCH, S. (1980) The SBAS: rationale, contents, scoring and reliability of a new interview schedule. *Social Psychiatry,* **15**, 43 – 55.

Quality of life

Quality of Life Schedule (QOL)
LEHMAN, A. (1983) The well being of chronic mental patients. *Archives of General Psychiatry*, **40**, 369 – 374.

Lancashire Quality of Life Profile
OLIVER, J. (1991) The social care directive: development of a quality of life profile for use in community services for the mentally ill. *Social Work & Social Sciences Review*, **3**, 5 – 45.

Physical health

Inputs such as annual physical check-ups might well result in improvement of the physical health of patients with long-term mental illness; this would also be a way of monitoring health.

Physical Health Index (PHI)
TEAM FOR THE ASSESSMENT OF PSYCHIATRIC SERVICES (1990) *Better Out Than In?* London: North East Thames Regional Health Authority.

Elderly service users (with dementia)

The Mini Mental State Examination (MMSE)
FOLSTEIN, M.F., FOLSTEIN, S.E. & McHUGH, P.O. (1975) "Mini-Mental State": a practical method for grading the cognitive state of patients for the clinician. *Journal of Psychiatric Research*, **12**, 189 – 198.

Modified Chrichton Royal Behavioural Rating Scale (MCRBRS)
WILKIN, D. & JOLLEY, D. (1979) *Behavioural Problems Among Old People in Geriatric Wards, Psychogeriatric Wards and Residential Homes.* Research report No.1, pp. 6 – 78. Manchester: Departments of Psychiatry & Community Medicine, University of Manchester.

Carers

General Health Questionnaire (GHQ)
GOLDBERG, D.P. (1972) *The Detection of Psychiatric Illness by Questionnaire.* Maudsley Monograph No. 21. London: Oxford University Press.

16 Community mental health

STEPHEN DORRELL

In April 1991, at the launch of the Centre for Mental Health Services Development, I described, in the words of the White Paper *Caring for People,* the Government's longstanding policy of developing locally based, community orientated, health and social services for people with psychiatric disorder as a "civilised and humanitarian one". I went on to say that "Virtually everyone concerned with mental health shares that view, whether sufferers, their families and carers, professional staff, or managers responsible for services". The international nature of this book indeed shows the worldwide movement towards, and commitment to community mental health services.

The policy of locally based community mental health services was first established in this country 30 years ago and has enjoyed continuing support from governments of both political parties, and from most professional staff working in the health services. Research funded by the Government shows that patients moved from old-style mental hospitals to comprehensive community programmes usually do well on transfer; that readmissions are generally short-term and rarely happen more than once, and that with a good district service, the majority of patients and their relatives are usually content, despite facing long-term problems. The evidence from such research both here and from abroad, particularly from the USA, strongly supports the conclusion that mentally ill people, including chronic and severe patients, can be successfully treated, in freedom, in the community.

Yet notwithstanding political support and sound policy, the build up of locally based services has been slower than many would like. Sometimes the quality of the community services provided has not always been adequate, and there have undoubtedly been cases where health and social service authorities have not been able to provide individual patients with the level of continuing health or social care in the community that was necessary. In parallel with this patchy development, and to a large extent underlying it, is the grotesque imbalance in the distribution of resources. There are approximately 40 000 patients in old long-stay hospitals consuming over half the mental health budget, whereas less than half the budget is available for the remaining hundreds of thousands of mentally ill people, most of whom are cared for in the community. The appropriate realignment of resources is a critical target for the development of community mental health services. Major improvements in community care for people with a psychiatric disorder could be achieved by using the existing resources more effectively; the encouragement of a more efficient use of resources by health authorities is a key function of this Centre for Mental Health Services Development.

In order to facilitate the transfer of resources into community care, the Government has introduced the Capital Loans Fund. This scheme provides bridging finance to assist Health Authorities replace outdated mental hospitals with modern, locally based facilities. The loans are to be repaid from the sale of the redundant sites. Over the two years of the scheme's existence, a total of £57 million has been committed to it so far. The Government has also taken specific action in an attempt to ensure that the needs of mentally ill people for health and social care are both systematically assessed and treated. Since April 1991, health authorities have been required to implement the care programme approach, which essentially promotes good professional practice. Each patient being considered for discharge, and all new patients accepted by the specialist psychiatric services are assessed in respect of their health and social care needs, including accommodation, and a decision is then made as to whether they can be viably treated in the community. If a patient's minimum requirements for community care cannot be met, then it is envisaged that in-patient care should be offered.

Treatment in the community is based upon a care programme which is drawn up after consultation with the multidisciplinary team, local authority social workers, general practitioners, the primary care team and, most importantly, with the agreement of the patients themselves and their carers.

Carers make a major and valued contribution to the support received by mentally ill people; indeed, the carers are by far the greatest natural resource we have in looking after people suffering from psychiatric illness. They often know a great deal about the patient's earlier life, previous interests, abilities, and contacts, and may have personal experience of the illness going back many years. Where a care programme depends on such a contribution it should be agreed in advance with the carer, who should be properly advised about the patient's condition, how to manage it, and how to obtain professional advice and support. The care programme also includes the nomination of a key worker to keep in close contact with the patient and to ensure that the agreed health and social care is in fact being delivered.

In order to support the implementation of the care programme approach, the Government has introduced the Mental Illness Specific Grant. This is paid directly to local authorities to assist in providing the social care element of the programme. In the financial year 1991 – 92 it was £20.2 million, and in the following year, 1992 – 93, it increased by 55% to £31.4 million to support expenditure of £44.9 million. In tandem with the Mental Illness Specific Grant, the Government has introduced supplementary credit approvals. These allow local authorities to finance the capital elements of the new social care services, funded by the Mental Illness Specific Grant. In 1991 – 92, the supplementary credit approval was £10 million, increased in the next financial year to £10.5 million.

The National Health Service and Community Care Act, passed in 1990, provides the legislative basis for the introduction of an internal market into the National Health Service and the development of community care. I am convinced that these reforms provide the only realistic prospect for developing good quality, locally based psychiatric services, for which both health and local authorities have responsibilities.

In their new role as purchasers of services, district health authorities will need to concentrate on assessing the health needs of their local populations, and on planning services which aim to meet those needs. Local authorities are undertaking a parallel exercise in respect of community care. The contractual nature of service provision is bringing together the purchasers, that is the health and local authorities on the one hand, and the providers on the other hand, in an explicit discussion about content, quantity, quality, and cost of services. It is hoped that the introduction of these four elements into basic contracts will form the basis for a general improvement in services, as the issues of service content and quality are dealt with even more explicitly.

In 1991 the Institute of Health at King's College, London, published their Prospectus and Business Plan for the Centre for Mental Health Services Development. It set out a twofold mission: firstly "to help authorities with the implementation of comprehensive, locally-based mental health services by providing long-term consultancy assistance"; secondly, "to contribute to the development of national policy from a base of accumulating experience of the successful development of specific local mental health services".

The Centre's work with a dozen health authorities and their

associated social services departments in five health regions has progressed well: preparatory work is complete in a number of districts, and plans for new services are in various stages of development. The Centre is now examining the processes which will be used to assist the authorities they are working with to implement those plans. Throughout these stages, a key aim is to bring the views and experiences of users to bear, which is crucial if the National Health Service is to achieve the standards set out recently by the Government in *The Patients Charter*.

The second part of the Centre's mission – to contribute to the development of policy from a base of accumulating experience – will clearly follow on from the first. This book provides evidence of the importance that the Centre attaches to this objective, but in addition, the Centre's Advisory Board is already identifying issues that require detailed study and recommendation. In particular, it has recognised the lack of management capacity available. The record of both health and local authorities in implementing community care has been generally poor; there has been a lack of progress, and a failure to gain the confidence of professionals involved. It is significant that only five district health authorities have so far developed a comprehensive network of mental health services which does not rely on an old-style mental hospital, and only two of these authorities have managed this transformation of their services within existing resources.

The international aspect of this book is important. The illnesses that beset people in Britain are essentially no different from those that occur among the populations of the USA, the Antipodes, our European partners, or other nations. Our systems for meeting people's health needs may differ greatly in their organisation and culture, but those needs are not so different. However fervently we may believe in our own National Health Service as an effective way of meeting such needs, it would be foolish to think that we cannot learn and improve from the experience of others. The international experts who were invited to participate in this book represent a formidable selection of people with something important in common: they share the vision to meet the mental health needs of their populations in a manner at least broadly compatible with the philosophy and principles of the Centre. That, in turn, is consistent with British government policy since 1975.

In January 1992, the Centre for Mental Health Services Development organised a meeting of international clinicians, managers and users to explore the setting up of an international organisation of people who are implementing major change and innovation in community mental health services. The need for such an organisation was clearly identified, and those present agreed to an international network being established under the umbrella of the Centre for Mental Health Services Development. This new initiative will greatly assist in developing cooperation and understanding among people from the different countries which are moving towards the same goal as the UK – of achieving the development of community mental health services.

Index

Compiled by LINDA ENGLISH